Current Challenges in Childbirth

Edited by Julio Elito Jr.

Published in London, United Kingdom

Current Challenges in Childbirth
http://dx.doi.org/10.5772/intechopen.98080
Edited by Julio Elito Jr.

Contributors
Francis Pebolo Pebalo, Jackline Ayikoru, Rajasri G. Yaliwal, Zilma Silveira Nogueira Reis, Roberta Maia de Castro Romanelli, Gabriela Silveira Neves, Birye Dessalegn Mekonnen, Chalachew Adugna Wubneh, Benjamin Joseph Nggada, María del Carmen Del Carmen Gangotena, Julio Elito Jr., Jorge Francisco Kuhn dos Santos

First published in London, United Kingdom, 2023 by IntechOpen
IntechOpen is the global imprint of INTECHOPEN LIMITED, registered in England and Wales, registration number: 11086078, 5 Princes Gate Court, London, SW7 2QJ, United Kingdom

British Library Cataloguing-in-Publication Data
A catalogue record for this book is available from the British Library

Additional hard and PDF copies can be obtained from orders@intechopen.com

Current Challenges in Childbirth
Edited by Julio Elito Jr.
p. cm.
Print ISBN 978-1-80355-714-4
Online ISBN 978-1-80355-715-1
eBook (PDF) ISBN 978-1-80355-716-8

Meet the editor

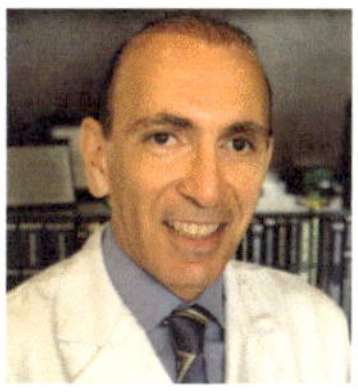

Julio Elito, Jr., Ph.D., obtained his master's degree and Ph.D. from the Federal University of São Paulo (UNIFESP), Brazil in 1995 and 1997, respectively. He is a specialist in laparoscopy and reproductive medicine. In 2006, he became an associate professor in the Department of Obstetrics, UNIFESP. He is currently head of the obstetrics discipline at the same university. Dr. Elito has published several journal articles and book chapters and has edited multiple books. He is a reviewer for several international journals and has presented at national and international congresses. He has been nominated as an "Honored Professor" several times by his students at the Medical School of UNIFESP.

Contents

Preface

Delivery assistance during childbirth is a major challenge today. Safety in childbirth to avoid maternal–fetal morbidity and mortality depends on proper usage of medications, avoiding early and unnecessary interventions, and limiting delays in decision-making. It is also important to consider the birthing person's expectations and desires. The setting where the delivery will occur should be prepared by a sensitive, respectful, and kind staff. It is important to avoid interventions such as fundal pressure, routine episiotomy, and unnecessary cesarean section. In addition, cultural and socioeconomic aspects as well as the patient's preferred birthing method are important factors in childbirth. The birthing person deserves an environment of respect without abusive measures.

This book presents important information on childbirth and stresses the importance of good-quality care. It covers the following topics: intrapartum care, induction of labor, episiotomy, uterotonics, new technologies to date pregnancy at birth, skin-to-skin contact, and contraception.

Chapter 1, "Introductory Chapter: Childbirth Challenges", is the introductory chapter and addresses the importance of respectful maternity care. Chapter 2, "Intrapartum Care: What Does the Evidence Say?", discusses labor progression, presenting information on the definition and duration of the latent and active first stages of labor and the progress of the first and second stages of labor. It also discusses pain relief during labor, prevention of postpartum hemorrhage (third stage of labor), and care of the newborn. Chapter 3, "Induction of Labour", describes the indications and contraindications for inducing labor, cervical repining, and induction agents and their complications. Chapter 4, "Update and Trend in Episiotomy Practice", evaluates the current trends in episiotomy, indications, obstetrical anal sphincter injuries (OASIS), and complications. Chapter 5, "Recent Advances in the Use of Uterotonics for the Prevention of Postpartum Hemorrhage", examines how to avoid postpartum hemorrhage, one of the leading causes of maternal morbidity and mortality. As such, the chapter describes various uterotonics. Chapter 6, "New Technologies to Dating Pregnancy at Birth", describes new methods of pregnancy dating at birth. Chapter 7, "Literacy on Skin-to-Skin Contact", discusses the importance of skin-to-skin contact in the care of the newborn. Finally, Chapter 8, " Utilization of Implant Contraceptive Methods and Associated Factors among Reproductive-Age Women in Ethiopia", discusses contraception.

I would like to thank my wife Camila and our children João and Pedro for their support, understanding, and love during the journey to complete this book.

Julio Elito Jr.
Associate Professor of the Department of Obstetrics,
Federal University of São Paulo (UNIFESP),
São Paulo, Brazil

Section 1

Introduction

Chapter 1

Introductory Chapter: Childbirth Challenges

Julio Elito Jr.

1. Introduction

Childbirth is one of the most important moments in life. Since the beginning, birth has always been surrounded by a fascination mixed with happiness and fear.

In medieval times, childbirth was a risky situation for both mother and baby. At that time, one in three women were victims of maternal mortality [1]. Infection, postpartum hemorrhage, obstructed labor, and poor knowledge of obstetrics were common causes of death [2].

Development of medicine and more detailed knowledge of the physiological process of childbirth brought safety. These aspects were essential to provide safer childbirth care by reducing maternal and perinatal mortality. The word Obstetrics derives from the Latin term "obstetrix", which is derived from the verb "obstare" (to be beside). This is the main mission of health professionals who embrace this specialty and accompany pregnant women at birth. Be at her side, fully supporting the parturient throughout the process and identifying risk situations that require intervention. "Obstare" (to be beside) is the motto that guides the specialty, and any act that opposes it can result in an avoidable error.

That is why the issue of childbirth care is so lively and current. Centuries passed, new knowledge was acquired, and behaviors were modified over time because they proved to be inefficient, and others were incorporated. Despite all development, we know that we live in a globalized world where different scenarios are presented, different socio-economic and cultural aspects that make birth a concern and several measures have been taken to reduce this distortion.

The United Nations among the goals for sustainable development stipulated, in 2016, some global strategies for the health of women, children, and adolescents. They listed three premises: survive, prosper, and transform [3].

One of the main strategies is the reduction of preventable deaths, among which are: reducing global maternal mortality to less than 70 deaths per 100,000 live births and reducing neonatal mortality to at least 12 per 1000 live births in all countries [3].

In addition, a very intense debate seeks to minimize obstetric care by dividing natural childbirth and cesarean section into two opposing groups. To relegate the importance of obstetrics to this dichotomy is to belittle the specialty. Obstetrics is much bigger than that. It involves the birth of a baby, a mother and a father.

Obstetrics is the specialty that receives the most complaints, as society considers childbirth a purely physiological event, without major complications. Thus, the pass away of a mother or a child represents, for the lay population, a disastrous performance of the assistance team, a situation in which technical knowledge is immediately questioned and, subsequently, it is considered malpractice and will be investigated by the medical board.

Childbirth care is a major challenge today. Safety in childbirth care to avoid maternal-fetal morbidity and mortality is especially important. However, there are still 810 maternal deaths per day from complications in pregnancy and childbirth, mostly from preventable or treatable causes such as infectious diseases, hemorrhage, pre-eclampsia, and complications during or after pregnancy and childbirth [4, 5].

It is essential to avoid, on the one hand, excessive medicalization with early and unnecessary interventions and, on the other hand, the lack of care that can lead to delays in decision-making. In this delicate balance, it is also important to consider the expectations of the parturient with her desires related to how the delivery she idealized will take place. Respecting their wishes without jeopardizing the maternal-fetal unit is a great challenge for the obstetrician. The scenario where the birth will take place must be prepared by a sensitive, respectful, and kind team. It is important to avoid interventions such as uterine pressure, routine episiotomy, and excess unnecessary cesarean sections. Cultural, socioeconomic aspects and the choice of delivery mode are part of a big puzzle.

This book aims to assess the best childbirth care within the scientific evidence. Good quality care is essential for maternal and fetal safety. The book will cover the following topics: intrapartum care, episiotomy, uterotonics, induction of labor, new technologies to date pregnancy at birth, skin-to-skin contact, and contraception.

The contribution of this book is to present the reader with scientific evidence on the topic of Childbirth. We believe that with initiatives like this we will be contributing to sustainable development with a reduction in maternal and neonatal mortality. The progress of a society is linked to conditions that provide women with safe motherhood and that culminate in the birth of a child with the right to physical and mental health.

The purpose of obstetrics is to preserve the integrity of maternal health and provide the unborn with all the promising potential for their full somatic, neurological, and psychological development, in order to become a healthy citizen physically and psychically. Thus, it will have the necessary conditions to be useful to society, and to the family, and will be able to dazzle a happy future.

Author details

Julio Elito Jr.
Department of Obstetrics, Federal University of São Paulo (UNIFESP), São Paulo, Brazil

*Address all correspondence to: elitojjr@hotmail.com

References

[1] Drife J. The start of life: A history of obstetrics. Postgraduate Medical Journal. 2002;**78**(919):311-315. DOI: 10.1136/pmj.78.919.311

[2] Say L, Chou D, Gemmill A, Tunçalp Ö, Moller AB, Daniels J, et al. Global causes of maternal death: A WHO systematic analysis. The Lancet Global Health. 2014;**2**(6):e323-e333. DOI: 10.1016/S2214-109X(14)70227-X

[3] The Global Strategy For Women's, Children's And Adolescents' Health (2016-2030) | Every Woman Every Child. Available from: https://globalstrategy.everywomaneverychild.org

[4] Trends in Maternal Mortality 2000 to 2017: Estimates by WHO, UNICEF, UNFPA, World Bank Group and the United Nations Population Division. Geneva: WHO; 2019 [cited 2020 November 10]. Available from: https://www.unfpa.org/sites/default/files/pub-pdf/Maternal_mortality_report.pdf

[5] Hoyert DL, Miniño AM. Maternal mortality in the United States: Changes in coding, publication, and data release, 2018. National Vital Statistics Reports. 2020;**69**(02):1-18

Section 2

Labour

Chapter 2

Intrapartum Care: What Does the Evidence Say?

Julio Elito Jr. and Jorge Francisco Kuhn dos Santos

Abstract

Childbirth is one of the most important moments in life. Delivery assistance is a major challenge today. Safety in childbirth care to avoid maternal-fetal morbidity and mortality is especially important. It is vital to avoid, on the one hand, the excess of medicalization with early and unnecessary interventions and, on the other hand, the lack of care that can lead to a delay in decision-making. In this delicate balance, it is also important to consider the expectation of the parturient with her desires related to how the birth she idealized will happen. Respecting her wishes without putting the maternal-fetal unity at risk is a great challenge for the obstetrician. It is important to avoid interventions as fundal pressure, routine episiotomy and the excess of unnecessary caesarean section. Cultural, socio-economical aspects and choosing the delivery mode are part of a big puzzle. This chapter aims to assess the best childbirth care among the scientific evidence and will cover the following topics: first stage of labor (differentiating latent from active phase), progression of the first and second stages of labor, pain relief during labor, prevention of postpartum hemorrhage, care of the newborn, and the puerperal woman.

Keywords: first stage of labour, second stage of labour, third stage of labour, postpartum haemorrhage, newborn

1. Introduction

In this chapter, the main care standards during labour and childbirth will be addressed. Several challenges related to labour assistance in the first, second and third stage will be presented based on the best scientific evidence.

2. First stage of labour

Delivery care begins with the correct diagnosis of first stage of labour: presence of at least two rhythmic and painful uterine contractions within 10 minutes, lasting around 30–50 seconds, with cervical changes.

An important point to consider is knowing how to differentiate the latent from the active phase of labour. In the latent phase, the parturient presents uterine contractions that cause changes in the process of effacement and dilation of the cervix, and this progression takes longer until reaching a dilation of 5 cm. On the other hand, in the active phase of the first stage of dilation of labour, the rhythm of uterine contractions is regular, and at this stage there is already significant cervical effacement and the dilation of the cervix progresses at an accelerated rate from 5 cm until complete dilation.

Hospitalisation is recommended during the period of the active first stage of labour. When in doubt, a period of observation should be done [1].

During the active first stage of labour, the patient is hospitalised, after anamnesis and general physical and obstetrical examination. Labour can take several hours—in general the primiparous, up to 15 hours and, in the multiparous, 10 hours. However, the duration of latent phase is more difficult to estimate. On the other hand, when cervical dilation is 5 cm, the mean duration of the first active stage is approximately 4 hours in primiparous and 3 hours in multiparous.

An important point to be considered regarding the first stage of labour is to avoid perform interventions, sometimes unnecessary, only considering the duration of the cervical dilatation period [2].

To avoid prolonged fasting during labour, pregnant women can drink fluids and eat light meals.

The parturient is instructed to take a bath with antiseptic soap and stimulated to empty the bowels if necessary. The administration of enema is not recommended.

Perineal and pubic shaving is not performed routinely.

The parturient is released so that she can adopt the position that seems most comfortable to her. When lying down, left lateral recumbency is preferable. Walking is allowed in the initial dilation and with an intact water bag. The parturient at this stage of labour should be encouraged to move, walking or exercising on the physiotherapy ball [3].

The presence of a companion chosen by the patient is allowed during labour and delivery [4]. On admission, in patients who did not undergo prenatal care or who were not undergoing obstetric ultrasound (US) during pregnancy, US is performed primarily with the aim of screening for major foetal malformations that have not been clinically detected.

It is essential to properly fill out the form of the partograph or WHO labour care guide, a simple and efficient graphic way of monitoring the work of childbirth. Its use facilitates the medical supervision of parturients and encourages partnership with obstetricians.

The concept that the average cervicodilation in primiparous women is approximately 1 cm per hour and, in multiparous women, it can reach 1.5 cm is unreliable to assess unfavourable evolution of labour. Therefore, several studies have shown that the partograph alert line cannot identify risk situations that can result in complications during childbirth.

In 2020, the WHO launched the Labour Care Guide to help health professionals use a more reliable instrument where they can record the main parameters of labour in order to find risk factors for adverse events in childbirth. Cervical dilatation, foetal heart rate, caput succedaneum, moulding, status of amniotic fluid, foetal descent, maternal temperature, blood pressure and urinary output should be recorded on the graph (**Figure 1**) [5]. The partograph should start from a cervical dilatation of 5 cm (active first stage of labour).

The digital vaginal examination must be repeated every 4 hours, depending on the stage of evolution, always checking, in addition to cervical conditions, as much information as possible: presentation, position and variety of position; height of the presentation; presence of plastic phenomena; and appearance of the liquid amniotic when the bag is ruptured.

Uterine dynamics should be periodic (every hour), correcting functional dystocia with appropriate manoeuvres and interventions if necessary. Surveillance of foetal

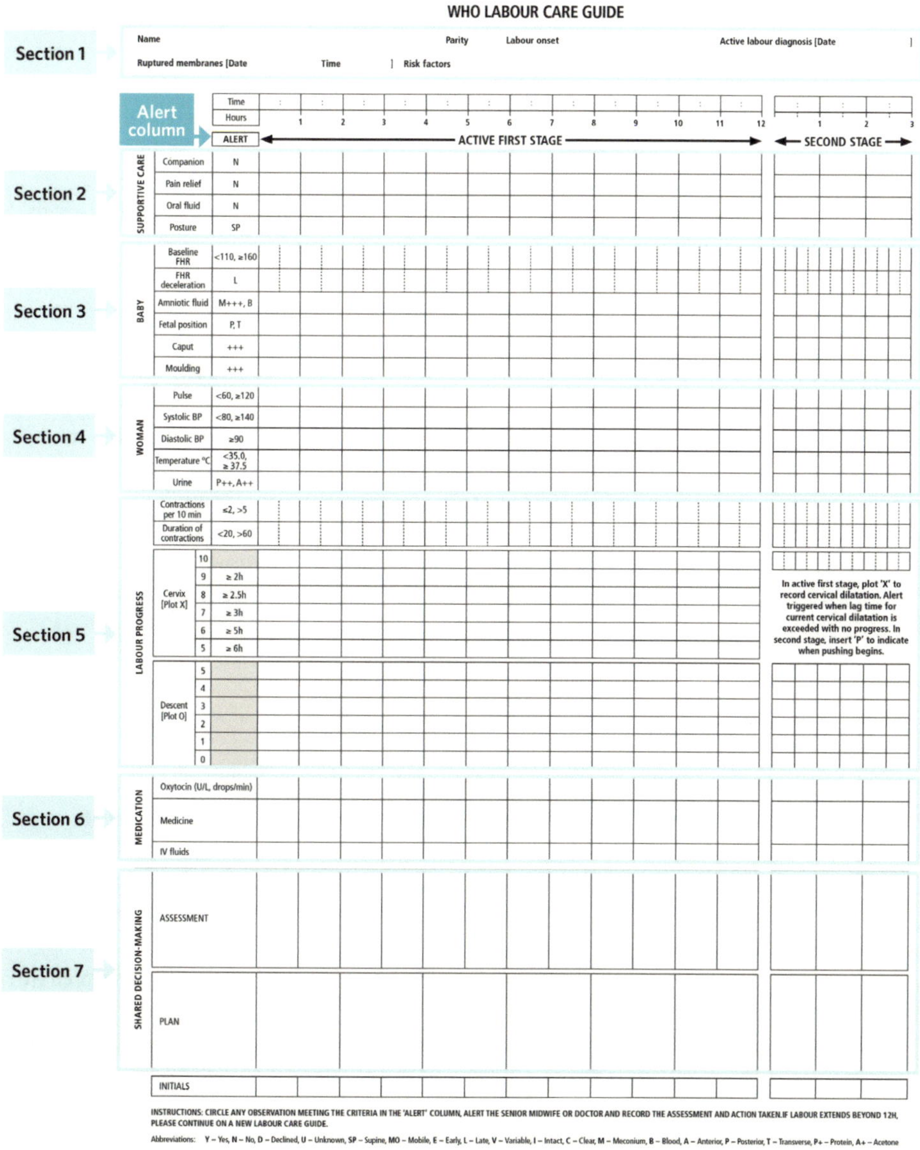

Figure 1.
WHO labour care guide [5].

well-being can be carried out intermittently in cases without pathologies, every 15–30 minutes by Doppler sonar. Often foetal heart rate should be assessed before, during and after uterine contraction for one or more minutes.

Cardiotocography should be used when there are changes during intermittent clinical auscultation of the foetal heart rate [6].

All interventions must be clearly described in the patient's medical record.

Pain relief during labour can be done by pharmacological or non-pharmacological measures. If the environment is favourable and there is a good interaction between the parturient and the care team, the focus on pain may be different. Initial pain relief measures are generally non-pharmacological. Among them we highlight: bath or hot compresses, massages in the lumbar region and relaxing breathing [7]. Several studies show that these measures are effective and the woman has a more positive experience related to childbirth. Among the pharmacological measures, epidural analgesia is the most used and best resolves pain. The use of opioids is a therapeutic alternative also used; however, it has side effects such as nausea, vomiting, drowsiness and even respiratory depression in the newborn [8].

Routine amniotomy is not recommended. If it is necessary to perform the amniotomy it should be done, with dilatation from 6 to 8 cm and fixed head, right after a contraction, in the most anterior portion possible, promoting slow flow of amniotic fluid and attention to its characteristics.

At the beginning of the expulsive period (complete cervicodilation), the parturient should be taken to the delivery room. Ideally, keep it in practically sitting position or, at least, with the trunk well raised.

Low foetal presentation, compressing the rectum and the perineum, determining the moment to perform the pulls, simultaneously with the contractions.

The main complication of the first stage is the cessation of labour. The diagnosis is made when the parturient is at least 6 cm dilated, has ruptured membranes and does not present any cervical changes due to at least 4 hours of adequate contractions or at least 6 hours of inadequate contractions with use of oxytocin to try to obtain adequate contractions [9].

3. Second stage of labour

The second stage of labour comprises the period between full cervical dilatation and the birth of the newborn. In this phase, the parturient performs involuntary pulls due to the uterine contractions of the expulsive period.

At this stage, the duration is variable. In primiparous women, this period can last up to 3 hours and in those from the second pregnancy onwards, the duration does not exceed 2 hours.

Maternity should be a welcoming environment, respecting ethical principles during childbirth care.

Auscultation of foetal heart rate with Doppler sonar or Pinard stethoscope should be performed every 5 minutes lasting 1 minute in the second stage of labour. This auscultation is performed during and after uterine contraction in order to observe whether there has been an acceleration or deceleration of the foetal heart rate.

The patient is free to choose the position that she feels most comfortable, such us upright, supine or other position [10]. Regardless of the chosen position, the care team must assess foetal well-being. If any deceleration is identified and there is a need to change position, the parturient must be clearly informed of the reason for this change. In the expulsive period of labour, the patient must be supported and encouraged to perform the pushing as she wishes [11].

During the expulsive period, some measures can be used to try to avoid perineal trauma, including perineal massage, the use of warm compresses on the perineum and protection of the perineum in the detachment of the cephalic pole [12].

Episiotomy should not be performed routinely [13].

The Kristeller manoeuvre, which consists of applying pressure to the uterine fundus in an attempt to shorten the expulsive period, is contraindicated due to the risks of maternal and foetal trauma [14].

The prolonged second stage of labour is generally defined as 2–3 hours for primiparous women and 1–2 hours for multiparous women, with the longest interval for women with epidural analgesia during labour [15]. In these situations, the risk of maternal morbidity increases, including postpartum complications such as infection and haemorrhage; it also increases the risk of perinatal morbidity.

4. Third stage of labour

Physiological delivery occurs approximately 5–10 minutes after foetal expulsion. If it does not occur after this period, it is called delayed delivery (up to 30 minutes) and placental retention (from 30 minutes).

The use of uterotonics in this stage for the prevention of postpartum haemorrhage is recommended. Oxytocin (10 IU IM/IV) is recommended as the first option. If oxytocin is not available or failure to prevent postpartum haemorrhage, the use of ergometrine/methylergometrine or oral misoprostol (600 μg) is recommended [16].

Delayed clamping of the umbilical cord is recommended after the first minute of life, with the aim of improving perinatal outcomes due to the increase in haemoglobin levels at birth, improvement of iron stores in the first months of life, reduction of rates of intraventricular haemorrhage and necrotizing enterocolitis in premature infants [16].

The prolonged third phase of labour increases the risk of postpartum bleeding. Placental complications of the third stage of labour include: retained placenta, adherent placenta and placenta accrete. Due to these complications, it may be necessary to perform the manual removal of the placenta, revision of the uterine cavity, massive bleeding requiring blood transfusion and even hysterectomy [17].

5. Care of the woman after birth

The period of 1 hour after delivery, also called the fourth period of labour or the Greenberg period, basically consists of careful monitoring by the obstetrician and the nursing team of the patient: in this period, bleeding can occur mainly, responsible for maternal mortality. Therefore, the volume of vaginal bleeding is the main parameter in command of how quickly important decisions must be made. Therefore, the assessment of uterine tone by postpartum abdominal palpation is the main measure for the early diagnosis of uterine atony. In addition, vaginal bleeding, uterine height, blood pressure and heart rate should be evaluated [18].

Breastfeeding in the first hour of life is recommended due to its importance for both the baby and the mother, as it helps with uterine contractions, reducing the risk of bleeding. And, in addition to health issues, breastfeeding strengthens the affective bond between mother and child [18].

6. Conclusions

The antenatal care is the start of preparation of a safe and quality care during childbirth. For a positive childbirth experience is mandatory a practice based on scientific evidence. Definition of latent and active first stage of labour is important for assistance. Active first stage starts when regular uterine contractions cause cervical effacement and cervical dilatation from 5 cm until full dilatation. Second stage is a challenge period and the duration varies: in first labour, birth is usually completed within 3 hours, whereas in subsequent labours, birth is usually completed within 2 hours. The use of uterotonics (oxytocin 10 U IM/IV) in the third stage for the prevention of postpartum haemorrhage is recommended.

Author details

Julio Elito Jr.* and Jorge Francisco Kuhn dos Santos
Department of Obstetrics, Federal University of São Paulo (UNIFESP), São Paulo, Brazil

*Address all correspondence to: elitojjr@hotmail.com

References

[1] Kobayashi S, Hanada N, Matsuzaki M, Takehara K, Ota E, Sasaki H, et al. Assessment and support during early labour for improving birth outcomes. Cochrane Database of Systematic Reviews. 2017;**4**:CD011516

[2] Wei S, Wo BL, Qi H-P, Xu H, Luo Z-C, Roy C, et al. Early amniotomy and early oxytocin for prevention of, or therapy for, delay in first stage spontaneous labour compared with routine care. Cochrane Database of Systematic Reviews. 2013;**8**:CD006794

[3] Lawrence A, Lewis L, Hofmeyr GJ, Styles C. Maternal positions and mobility during first stage labour. Cochrane Database of Systematic Reviews. 2013;**10**:CD003934

[4] Bohren MA, Hofmeyr GJ, Sakala C, Fukuzawa RK, Cuthbert A. Continuous support for women during childbirth. Cochrane Database of Systematic Reviews. 2017;**7**:CD003766

[5] WHO Labour Care Guide: User's Manual. Geneva: World Health Organization; 2020. Licence: CC BY-NC-SA 3.0 IGO

[6] Devane D, Lalor JG, Daly S, McGuire W, Cuthbert A, Smith V. Cardiotocography versus intermittent auscultation of fetal heart on admission to labour ward for assessment of fetal wellbeing. Cochrane Database of Systematic Reviews. 2017;**1**:CD005122

[7] Smith CA, Levett KM, Collins CT, Crowther CA. Relaxation techniques for pain management in labour. Cochrane Database of Systematic Reviews. 2011;**12**:CD009514

[8] Anim-Somuah M, Smyth RM, Jones L. Epidural versus non-epidural or no analgesia in labour. Cochrane Database of Systematic Reviews. 2011;**12**:CD000331

[9] Spong CY, Berghella V, Wenstrom KD, et al. Preventing the first cesarean delivery: Summary of a joint Eunice Kennedy Shriver National Institute of Child Health and Human Development, Society for Maternal-Fetal Medicine, and American College of Obstetricians and Gynecologists workshop. Obstetrics & Gynecology. 2012;**120**(5):1181-1193

[10] Gupta J, Sood A, Hofmeyr G, Vogel J. Position in the second stage of labour for women without epidural anaesthesia. Cochrane Database of Systematic Reviews. 2017;**5**:CD002006

[11] Lemos A, Amorim MM, Dornelas de Andrade A, de Souza AI, Cabral Filho JE, Correia JB. Pushing/bearing down methods for the second stage of labour. Cochrane Database of Systematic Reviews. 2017;**3**:CD009124

[12] Aasheim V, Nilsen ABV, Reinar LM, Lukasse M. Perineal techniques during the second stage of labour for reducing perineal trauma. Cochrane Database of Systematic Reviews. 2017;**6**:CD006672

[13] Jiang H, Qian X, Carroli G, Garner P. Selective versus routine use of episiotomy for vaginal birth. Cochrane Database of Systematic Reviews. 2017;**2**:CD000081

[14] Hofmeyr G, Vogel J, Cuthbert A. Fundal pressure during the second stage of labour. Cochrane Database of Systematic Reviews. 2017;**3**:CD006067

[15] NICE. Intrapartum Care. Care of Healthy Women and Their Babies during Childbirth. NICE Clinical Guidelines. London: NICE; 2007. p. 55

[16] WHO Recommendations: Intrapartum Care for a Positive Childbirth Experience. Geneva: World Health Organization; 2018. Licence: CC BY-NC-SA 3.0 IGO

[17] Rotem R, Lipski A, Weintraub AY, Baumfeld Y, Yohay D, Press F, et al. Third stage of labor placental complications and placenta-associated syndromes. The Journal of Maternal-Fetal & Neonatal Medicine. Oct 2021;**34**(20):3350-3354

[18] Cunningham FG, Leveno KJ, Dashe JS, Hoffman BL, Spong CY, Casey BM. Phisiology of labor. In: Cunningham FG, Leveno KJ, Dashe JS, Hoffman BL, Spong CY, Casey BM, editors. Williams Obstetrics. 26th ed. New York: McGraw-Hill; 2022. p. 1030

Chapter 3

Induction of Labour

Benjamin Joseph Nggada

Abstract

Induction of labour is one of the common obstetric interventions in the world with varied incidence rates between developed and developing countries. It is generally employed by obstetricians and physicians managing pregnant women when the risk of continuing such pregnancy is far greater than delivery at that said point. A detailed evaluation and indications for induction of labour should be done for every single woman. Methods of induction of labour could be pharmacological, mechanical or both; taking care to reduce or eliminate complications associated with this intervention. Decision for induction of labour should involve the most senior member of the team with a woman centered approach to care. Induction of labour carries multiple risks and complications compared with spontaneous onset of uterine contractions with increase tendency of operative vaginal delivery and caesarean section.

Keywords: pre-inductive cervical state, induction of labour, onset of labour, postdate, augmentation, misoprostol

1. Introduction

Induction of Labour (IOL) is one of the common obstetric procedures and or intervention encountered in maternity unit(s) all over the world [1]. Usually, the risk of continued pregnancy is far more detrimental to the mother or her unborn baby or both [1, 2]. Therefore, a balance in favour delivery is anticipated and planned with the anticipating mother using a woman centered approach [3, 4]. Decision for induction of labour should be led by the most experienced obstetrician on ground in consultation with the team managing such pregnancy. IOL will set up a cascade of events cumulating to the delivery of the baby and automatically elevates that pregnancy state to high risk [2]. These processes are important that they are closely monitored to end point and beyond.

2. Epidemiology

The incidence of induction of labour varies between different settings and appears to be on the rise especially in developed countries. In the United States the rate of IOL is quoted to be approximately 30 percent [5]. While in the United Kingdom (UK) the recent maternity figures show an increase rate of 2.1% from the 29.4% in 2016–2017 to 31.6% in 2017–2018 [6] according to the Hospital Episode Statistics. This increase in induction rates in developed countries and particularly in the UK is attributed to improved diagnostic tools and better understanding of maternal medicine, advanced maternal age, and socioeconomic class variation [7–9]. The incidence of induction in Africa has been found to be below 10 percent in most settings. In a recent cross-sectional study to assess the prevalence, outcome and associated factors among women delivered at public hospitals in Ethiopia, Lueth et al. [10] reported a prevalence of 9% and failed IOL was responsible for 3.3% increase in caesarean section rates. Vogel et al. [11] in a secondary analysis of data for World Health Organization (WHO) global survey on maternal and neonatal health found that the unmet needs of IOL were between 60% and 80% with an average rate of IOL of 4.4%. In resource-constrained settings there is less capacity due to inadequate facilities, lack of trained staff and limited centers where safe caesarean sections can be performed on a 24 h basis.

3. Definition of terms

In order to understand the concept of induction of labour, some key terms need to be clearly understood:

Induction of Labour (IOL): This refers to the artificial initiation of uterine contractions before their spontaneous onset at or beyond the age of viability with the sole aim of delivery of the fetoplacental unit where the benefit of pregnancy termination exceeds its prolongation [1, 2, 7, 10, 11].

Successful IOL: Is said to occur when vaginal delivery is achieved usually within 24–48 h [12].

Failed IOL: In recent National Institute for Health and Care Excellence (NICE) guideline, unsuccessful IOL is considered when once cycle of treatment has failed to initiate uterine contractions [13]. Some authors refer to failed induction as the inability to achieved adequate uterine contractions after 6–8 h of oxytocin administration and at ceiling doses for at least an hour [14]. It is important to understand that failed IOL should not always results in emergency caesarean section as studies have shown that considerable number of women will delivery beyond such set points [15].

Cervical ripening: Is the change of cervical physical and chemical (intrinsic) morphology as a result of realignment of collagen fibres and extracellular matrix from firm to a compliant structure with gradual softening, effacement and dilatation which increases the likelihood of vaginal delivery. It can be from a natural process, chemically or mechanically induced [12, 13, 16].

Tachysystole: Is said to occur when there are greater than 5 contractions in 10 min in a period of approximately 30 min. Uterine tachysystole is further subdivided into two categories: with or without fetal heart rate changes [13, 17–19]. This could be spontaneous or induced.

Hypertonus: When uterine contractions duration is more than 2 min without fetal heart rate changes. This is also considered as increase in uterine tonus, which is intrauterine pressure between contractions [13, 19].

Hyperstimulation: Refers to tachysystole or hypertonus with abnormal fetal heart rate changes. This term is largely abandoned, and it is replaced with tachysystole with fetal heart abnormalities. [13, 18].

4. Understanding onset of labour

Labour diagnosis is one of the most important clinical judgements in maternity care and is much more important to understand its onset. However, the mechanisms involved in the onset of labour still remains blurred and why some women will reach postdate or post term without spontaneous onset of labour is elusive. Our narrow understanding of the mechanism of onset of labour makes IOL difficult [19]. Usually, a cascade of biochemical events heralds the onset of a complex well-regulated process that results in cervical ripening, occasional membrane rupture and high frequency myometrial contraction that result in the expulsion of the fetoplacental unit [20].

The mechanism of spontaneous onset of labour has a fetal, placental/fetal membranes and maternal components that contribute to its onset via series of paracrine/autocrine hormones. Uterine quiescence that is maintained throughout pregnancy is switched off by the withdrawal of the functional inhibitory effect of progesterone via progesterone receptor (PR). There is an increase unbalance ratio of progesterone receptor key isoforms with more expression of progesterone receptor A (PR-A) compared with progesterone receptor B (PR-B) that increases with advancing gestational age and might also inhibit the PR-B genes. The overwhelming increased ratio of PR-A to PR-B may promote transcription of contractile protein CX43 [20, 21] and increase gap junctions' formation in the myometrium [22]. Oxytocin receptors (OXTR) gradually increase with advancing gestational age which may directly increase intracellular calcium concentrations [23].

Prostaglandins (PG) play major roles in initiation and maintenance of uterine contraction via prostaglandin receptors. The prostaglandins that play major role in inducing myometrial contractility are prostaglandin E2 (PGE2) and prostaglandin F2α (PGF2α) which induces intracellular calcium by opening calcium gated channels. Spontaneous labour is also associated with sterile inflammation with increase infiltration of leucocytes and upregulation of inflammatory cytokines and chemokines, particularly interleukin 1B which increases expression of calcium transport protein. Though there are plethora of literatures toward the physiology of the onset of labour, its exact pathway remains elusive [20–23].

5. Indications and contraindications of IOL

The indication(s) for induction of labour should be weighed on the scale of clinical judgement to ascertain that the benefit(s) of delivery outweighs continuation or prolongation of such pregnancy (**Table 1**). This decision should be taken seriously, and there should be shared decision between the managing clinicians and the woman as well as appropriate informed consent taken. Prior to informed consent there should be a dialogue on the primary indication for IOL and other contributory factors, risks and benefits, methods and rationale, and realistic expectations [24].

6. Preinduction cervical state

The Bishop's score is used to assess the pre-inductive state of the cervix and to forecast the favorability of the cervix to comply during IOL. IOL is highly likely to fail if it is embarked upon without a proper assessment of the woman and consideration of the bishop score. The cervix retains its firm rigidity throughout pregnancy. As the uterus enlarges, the cervix becomes softer and distensible in preparation for labour and delivery by ripening. Ripening is a complex series of biochemical processes that results in softening of the cervix, effacement, and dilation. This usually occurs prior to uterine contractions for both spontaneous and iatrogenic labour. The cervix is composed of fibroid connective tissue, collagen (type I, III predominately and a small amount of type IV), elastin, vasculature, fibroblast, and smooth muscle [25, 26].

Indications [13, 25]	Contraindications [13, 25]] confirmed
Post term >42 weeks	Maternal refusal
Late term pregnancy/postdate 41 0–41 6 weeks	Prior classical, De Lee or inverted T incision
Preeclampsia >37 weeks	Significant prior uterine surgery (e.g. full thickness myomectomy)
Eclampsia	
Chronic hypertension	Previous hysterotomy
Gestational hypertension >38 weeks	Two or more previous caesarean sections
Twin gestation	
• Uncomplicated dichorionic twin pregnancy > 38 weeks	Previous uterine rupture
• Uncomplicated monochorionic twin pregnancy > 36/37 weeks	Fetal malpresentation (e.g. transverse lie, footling breech)
Diabetes in pregnancy or gestational diabetes	
Alloimmune disease near term or at term	Placenta previa
IUGR	Vasa previa
IUFD	Cord presentation
Intrahepatic cholestasis of pregnancy	Active genital herpes
Prelabour rupture of membrane at term or near term	Invasive cervical cancer
Preterm Prelabour rupture of membrane with GBS colonisation	
Oligohydramnios	
Chorioamnionitis	
Significant but stable antepartum haemorrhage	
Obstetric Cholestasis	
Controversial	
Prior IUFD	Previous vesicovaginal fistula
Care giver or maternal request	Previous OASIS
Suspected fetal macrosomia	
One previous caesarean section	

Table 1.
Indication for induction of labour.

Cervical remodelling is associated with increase vascularity, stromal and glandular hypertrophy. There is concomitant increase in inflammatory activities with production of cytokines which leads to the release of metalloproteases (2 and 9) that degrades cervical collagens. The extracellular matrix which is strengthened by proteoglycans is gradually reduced with an unbalanced increase in glycosaminoglycans. The remodelling of the cervix is associated with decreased cross-linkages between collagen helices which cumulates to increased compliance to softening, effacement, and dilation [26].

Various hormones are responsible for this complex interaction that leads to cervical ripening. Increase in cyclooxygenase −2 lead to rise in the level of local PGE2 and PGF2α. PGE2 will activate a series of reactions: increase dilatation of small vessels in the cervix, increase collagen degradation, increase in hyaluronic acid, increase chemotaxis for leucocytes and increase release of Interleukin −8. PGF2α stimulate an increase in glycosaminoglycans. The role of Nitric Oxide (NO) has been the focus on recent studies on its contribution to cervical ripening. Increased levels of induced Nitric Oxide Synthase (iNOS) activity by resident and migrating inflammatory cells is associated with cervical ripening by dramatic increase in NO. NO might play a role by increased activities of metalloproteases [27–29].

Dr. Edward Bishop in 1964 proposed a Prelabour scoring system to assess the likelihood of going into spontaneous labour [30]. It has now undergone several

Cervical features	Score			
	0	1	2	3
Cervical dilatation (cm)	0	1–2	3–4	>4
Length (cm)	>4	3–4	1–2	<1
Station of the presenting part (cm)	−3	−2	−1/0	+1/+2
Consistency	Firm	Average	Soft	—
Position	Posterior	Mid/Anterior	—	—

Table 2.
Modified Bishop's (Calder) score [31, 32] confirmed.

modifications to assess the favourability prior to IOL. The score is an aggregate sum of the cervical dilatation, consistency, effacement, position and fetal station [31]. A total score of 6 and above is considered favourable and score below that is deemed unfavourable. The Calder Modification replaces cervical effacement with cervical length with a total score of 12 (**Table 2**) [31, 32]. In a retrospective study [33] done recently to closely look at the relationship between bishop score and successful induction, a higher bishop score (8–10) at the beginning of IOL is directly proportional to the higher rates of successful IOL compared with bishop score between 6 and 7. There is recent evidence to show that the cervical length assessment by transvaginal ultrasound appear to be superior to the bishop score, however this is not a routine practice [34].

7. IOL check list

An induction check list is good clinical practice to ensure women are properly prepared, improve IOL success and prevent complications. Every maternity setting should have an IOL check list tailored to meet their local standard. A check list should have the patient's biodata, informed consent, gestational age, indication for IOL, patient routine booking investigations, associated comorbidity, previous surgeries, and the bishop score. A recent ultrasound with estimated fetal weight - which also rules out any contraindication for vaginal delivery, an admission CTG and the method of cervical ripening and IOL with the responsible doctor's name and signature should be clearly documented [35].

8. Cervical ripening and IOL agents

Cervical ripening and induction agents can be group into pharmacological, mechanical and combination of both. While some agents are intended to ripen the cervix before initiation of induction of labour, majority will progress to initiate uterine contractions (see **Table 3**).

8.1 Prostaglandins

Prostaglandins have gained wide acceptance as a cervical ripening and induction agent over the decade and is now considered a preferred agent for both. However, they are said to be associated with a small risk for tachysystole and fetal heart rate changes [36]. Misoprostol—a synthetic prostaglandin E1 analogue—is heat stable and low cost

Pharmacological	Mechanical	Combination
Prostaglandins • Prostaglandin E2 (Dinoprostone) • Prostaglandin E1 (Misoprostol) Oxytocin	Transcervical catheters • Foley • Cook Extra-amniotic saline infusion Stripping membrane Laminaria Cervical hygroscopic dilators Extra-amniotic saline infusion	Transcervical catheter + Prostaglandins Transcervical catheter + Oxytocin

Table 3.
Cervical ripening and induction agents.

compared to Dinoprostone. This has seen its wide usage especially in low resource setting. Misoprostol availability is said to bring equity in the disparity of induction of labour between developed and resource constrained regions of the world and recently a low dose misoprostol preparation was approved for IOL in Nordic countries [37, 38]. The dosing and timing of misoprostol ranges 25–50 mcg every 2–6 h. However, in a study of balancing efficacy and safety, the minimum efficacious dose associated with less complication is 25 mcg [38], while the vaginal compared with the oral route appears to offer significant clinical advantage in successful vaginal delivery [39].

Dinoprostone is prostaglandin E2 that comes in two popular preparations as Cervidil, a control release hydrogel suppository 10 mg vaginal inserted every 12 h at 0.3 mg/h. and Prepidil administered as an intracervical gel of 0.5 mg/2.5 ml or 1 or 2 mg for intravaginal insertion every 4–6 h with a maximum of 3 doses in 24 h. Dinoprostone needs to be refrigerated and is relatively expensive for resource constrained settings [40, 41]. The International Federation of Obstetrics and Gynaecology (FIGO) recently established an expanded chart on the dosage of misoprostol in variety of Obstetric and Gynaecologic conditions in the light of new evidence and through expert contributions which has been endorsed by FIGO safe motherhood and newborn health committee (**Table 4**) [42].

8.2 Oxytocin

Oxytocin is a neuropeptide hormone produced by the hypothalamus via the paraventricular nuclei and stored in the posterior pituitary gland. It is secreted when triggered by labour, lactation, social interaction, and stressors. Oxytocin acts on the myometrium to induce uterine contractions via G-proteins with the subsequent release of intracellular calcium stores through a complex interplay on its activity on phospholipase C. Its potency is directly proportional with advancing gestational age when there are sufficient oxytocin receptors [43]. The synthetic oxytocin is a cyclic nonapeptide which is identical to the natural oxytocin obtained via chemical synthesis. Oxytocin acts within a minute of intravenous injection and 2–4 min via the intramuscular route. In a low dose infusion, it causes rhythmic uterine contractions with a repetitive pattern. It can cause sustained uterine contraction at high dose infusion. It reaches its steady state between 20 and 40 min during continuous infusion, and it is metabolised and cleared by the liver and kidneys with about 1 percent unchanged in the urine [43, 44].

Oxytocin might have plausible synergistic effect in cervical ripening, however its role as a cervical ripening agent is not well established [45]. There are still controversies on its optimal regimen for induction of labour with varied protocols in different settings. However, a low dose regimen initiated between 0.5 and 1 mU, and increased

FIGO
www.figo.org

MISOPROSTOL-ONLY RECOMMENDED REGIMENS 2017

<13 weeks' gestation	13–26 weeks' gestation	>26 weeks' gestation[8]	Postpartum use
Pregnancy termination[a,b,1] 800μg sl every 3 hours *or* pv*/bucc every 3–12 hours (2–3 doses)	**Pregnancy termination**[1,5,6] 13–24 weeks: 400μg pv*/sl/bucc every 3 hours[a,e] 25–26 weeks: 200μg pv*/sl/bucc every 4 hours[f]	**Pregnancy termination**[1,5,9] 27–28 weeks: 200μg pv*/sl/bucc every 4 hours[f,g] >28 weeks: 100μg pv*/sl/bucc every 6 hours	**Postpartum hemorrhage (PPH) prophylaxis**[i,2,10] 600μg po (x1) *or* **PPH secondary prevention**[j,11] (approx. ≥350ml blood loss) 800μg sl (x1)
Missed abortion[c,2] 800μg pv* every 3 hours (x2) *or* 600μg sl every 3 hours (x2)	**Fetal death**[f,g,1,5,6] 200μg pv*/sl/bucc every 4–6 hours	**Fetal death**[2,9] 27–28 weeks: 100μg pv*/sl/bucc every 4 hours[f] >28 weeks: 25μg pv* every 6 hours *or* 25μg po every 2 hours[h]	**PPH treatment**[k,2,10] 800μg sl (x1)
Incomplete abortion[a,2,3,4] 600μg po (x1) *or* 400μg sl (x1) *or* 400–800μg pv* (x1)	**Inevitable abortion**[a,2,3,5,6,7] 200μg pv*/sl/bucc every 6 hours	**Induction of labor**[h,2,9] 25μg pv* every 6 hours *or* 25μg po every 2 hours	
Cervical preparation for surgical abortion[d] 400μg sl 1 hour before procedure *or* pv* 3 hours before procedure	**Cervical preparation for surgical abortion**[a] 13–19 weeks: 400μg pv 3–4 hours before procedure >19 weeks: needs to be combined with other modalities		

References
- a WHO Clinical practice handbook for safe abortion, 2014
- b von Hertzen et al. Lancet, 2007; Sheldon et al. 2016 FIAPAC abstract
- c Gemzell-Danielsson et al. IJGO, 2007
- d Sääv et al. Human Reproduction, 2015; Kapp et al. Cochrane Database of Systematic Reviews, 2010
- e Dabash et al. IJGO, 2015
- f Perritt et al. Contraception, 2013
- g Mark et al. IJGO, 2015
- h WHO recommendations for induction of labour, 2011
- i FIGO Guidelines: Prevention of PPH with misoprostol, 2012
- j Raghavan et al. BJOG, 2015
- k FIGO Guidelines: Treatment of PPH with misoprostol, 2012

Notes
1. If mifepristone is available (preferable), follow the regimen prescribed for mifepristone + misoprostol[a]
2. Included in the WHO Model List of Essential Medicines
3. For incomplete/inevitable abortion women should be treated based on their uterine size rather than last menstrual period (LMP) dating
4. Leave to take effect over 1–2 weeks unless excessive bleeding or infection
5. An additional dose can be offered if the placenta has not been expelled 30 minutes after fetal expulsion
6. Several studies limited dosing to 5 times; most women have complete expulsion before use of 5 doses, but other studies continued beyond 5 and achieved a higher total success rate with no safety issues
7. Including ruptured membranes where delivery indicated
8. Follow local protocol if previous cesarean or transmural uterine scar
9. If only 200μg tablets are available, smaller doses can be made by dissolving in water (see www.misoprostol.org)
10. Where oxytocin is not available or storage conditions are inadequate
11. Option for community based programs

Route of Administration
pv – vaginal administration
sl – sublingual (under the tongue)
po – oral
bucc – buccal (in the cheek)

* Avoid pv (vaginal route) if bleeding and/or signs of infection

Rectal route is not included as a recommended route because the pharmacokinetic profile is not associated with the best efficacy

Table 4.
FIGO misoprostol-only recommended regimens 2017 [42] confirmed.

by 1 mU/min every 30–40 min interval is preferred over high dose regimen of 4–6 mU [44].

Maternal and Child Health (Obstetrics and Gynaecology Division) University of Namibia

A. Dosage

The dose of oxytocin is calculated using the formula: 10 units of oxytocin in 1000 ml of normal saline or ringers' lactate is equivalent to 10,000 mU. Therefore, each ml (1 ml) of fluid mix is 10 mU. In 1000 ml give 6 ml/h (60 mU/h.)

Starting dose at 1 mU/min oxytocin infusion should be escalated at 30 min interval until adequate and strong contractions (3–4 lasting 40–50 s in 10 min) is established.

The 2 IU in 200 ml is recommended because it is cost effective with less water intoxication in resource constrained settings. Oxytocin dose of greater than 20 mU/min highlighted in red is to be administered only by a senior resident doctor or a specialist. Low dose oxytocin infusion should be administered by infusion pump, however in settings where there are no infusion pumps, a senior doctor should closely monitor the infusion at a rate of 10 drops/min in a diluent of concentration of 10 IU in 1000 ml escalated every 30 min maximum of 60 drops/min.

B. Preparation

1. Obtain informed consent for oxytocin induction and or augmentation of labour

2. Do a pre induction and or augmentation CTG before the onset of oxytocin

3. Continuous CTG is advised for all patients

4. Do haemoglobin and obtain blood for blood group and save serum

5. Do not administer oxytocin on a previous uterine scar except by a specialist instruction (such specialist should monitor the patient)

6. Clearly document the indication for oxytocin use in the labour care guide

7. Inform all the managing/incoming team/theatre staff/Anaesthetist

8. For induction of labour: use oxytocin only in patients with bishop score >6 and perform artificial rupture of membrane if the membranes are intact

9. Do not give oxytocin within 6 h of prostaglandin use

C. Monitoring

1. Continuous CTG

2. Escalate the dosage every 30 min after assessment of maternal condition, fetal condition, and uterine contraction

3. Maintain, reduce, or stop dose when adequate uterine contractions are achieved (3–4 contractions in 10 min lasting 40–50 s)

4. Use the labour care guide in monitoring all patients on oxytocin infusion

5. STOP oxytocin and give plain normal saline whenever there is uterine hyperactivity:

   a. Tachysystole

   b. Hypertonus

   c. Hyperstimulation

The woman should adopt a left lateral position.

Consider supplemental oxygen, especially when there are signs of maternal hypoxia or category III CTG changes characterised by absent baseline variability with any of the following: recurrent late decelerations, recurrent variable decelerations, bradycardia, or sinusoidal pattern. Consider delivery if fetal heart rate abnormality persists.

6. Fetal rate abnormality may be the earliest sign of uterine rupture especially in patients on oxytocin infusion

7. After 4 h, stop infusion to reassess if there is any benefit of further infusion

8.3 Transcervical catheters

The transcervical extra-amniotic catheters have been one of the oldest methods of cervical ripening and induction of labour [46]. The Foley catheter has a single balloon with a capacity between 30 and 80 ml that is inserted into the extra-amniotic space compared to the more recent Cook's catheter with double balloons with one inserted into the extra-amniotic space as the uterine balloon and another below the cervix as the vaginal balloon with capacity of 80 ml for both [47]. In a Cochrane data base of systematic review of 23 studies [48], there were no statistically significant difference in comparing Foley catheter and prostaglandins in achieving vaginal delivery within 24 h with similar incidence of caesarean section rates. However, the transcervical Foley's catheter had lower incidence of tachysystole and or fetal heart rate abnormalities [48].

In a randomised controlled trial comparing a 30 and 80 ml Foley catheter balloon for preinduction cervical ripening, 80 ml provided faster labour, more dilatation and decrease need for oxytocin [49]. However, no significant difference was found between 12- and 24-h duration in induction delivery interval [46]. Other additives like applying traction and weight to the catheter has demonstrated faster expulsion of the Foley without any effect on the induction delivery interval (**Figure 1**) [50].

A single transcervical Foley catheter without extra-amniotic saline has better patient satisfaction with less discomfort compared with the double balloon catheter and it is cost effective especially in resource constrained settings [51]. Recent evidence is suggesting that highly motivated women can use transcervical Foley balloon in an outpatient setting with no increase in morbidity and or adverse outcome [52].

One of the major concerns of transcervical balloon catheters is theoretical risk of infection. This risk has not been validated and the rates of puerperal and neonatal infection appear similar to other methods of induction [53–55].

Combination of mechanical and pharmacologic methods has been one of the recent advances in labour induction to increase efficiency and efficacy, reduce cost and reduce adverse effects of induction agents to the mother and her baby. The BIGIN trial was a randomised control trial that compared buccal versus vaginal misoprostol

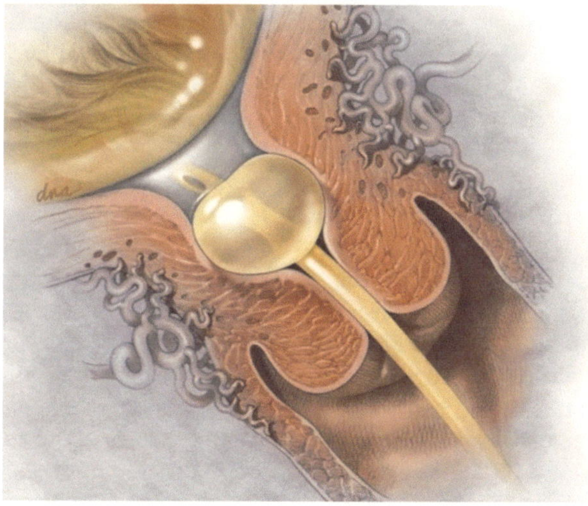

Figure 1.
Transcervical extra-amniotic Foley's catheter [46].

with Foley catheter. The vaginal misoprostol with Foley catheter resulted in a shorter induction delivery time with similar caesarean section rates, perinatal and maternal morbidity among both arms of the study. Therefore, vaginal misoprostol combination is recommended as the preferred method for combination method [56].

8.4 Stripping membrane

This is an old but reliable method of inducing cervical remodelling to comply with induction of labour. It is a mechanical method that involves a digital vaginal examination with the aim of placing one or two gloved fingers -usually the index and the middle - into the cervix and thereafter performing a circular sweeping motion. This is an artificial separation of the membrane that increases the activity of PGF2 and phospholipase which induces the complex cascade of cervical ripening [57]. In a recent Cochrane review [58], there is more likelihood to have spontaneous vaginal delivery among women who had their membranes swept. NICE guidelines on IOL recognised sweeping of membrane as an adjunct to formal induction [13]. Membrane sweeping can be offered to women from 39 weeks of gestation and thereafter additional membrane sweep could be offered at 40 and 41 weeks if there is no onset of spontaneous labour after the first membrane sweep [13]. There are concerns on the possibility of large doses of bacteria pushed above the internal os resulting in increased risk of maternal and fetal infection especially when there is a prolonged delay between membrane sweep and the onset of labour [57]. The role of cervical massage as an alternative method to membrane sweeping appears promising with significant effect on bishop score and can be considered as a reasonable option; especially if the cervical os is closed [59].

8.5 Laminaria and cervical hygroscopic dilators

Laminaria are dried seaweed stems (Laminaria japonica or Laminaria digitalis) that can be placed in the cervix to induce cervical ripening by absorbing water and expanding to cause cervical dilation and provoke endogenous prostaglandin release [60, 61]. Dilapan-S (MEDICEM, the Netherlands) is a sterile hygroscopic cervical dilator that has demonstrated no increased risk of infection like the laminaria tents. They are polymer rods which consist of the dilating part made of hydrogel and a polypropylene handle. An international observation study has revealed that Dilapan-S has not increased the risk of hyperstimulation and may be used in an outpatient setting [61, 62].

8.6 Artificial rupture of membranes (AROM)

Amniotomy can be used as an adjunct to induction of labour in a woman whose cervix is accessible and favourable. It is usually a prelude to oxytocin induction. However, in recent NICE guideline, it is not recommended as a sole method of induction with or without oxytocin except where prostaglandins are contraindicated [13, 61]. A recent randomised controlled trial has found that immediate oxytocin administration after AROM was not associated with shorter AROM to delivery time compared to delay of 4 h. Therefore, the decision to use any method should follow local protocols based on resources and maternal choice [63]. It is important to remember that there is a major risk of the cord prolapse with an unengaged presenting part.

Other methods of cervical ripening and induction of labour are yet to be clinically validated. Therefore, the use of mifepristone, acupuncture, homoeopathy, hypnotic relaxation, baths, enema, sexual intercourse, breast stimulation, intracervical hyaluronidase, relaxin, corticosteroids, and oestrogen need further research [64].

9. IOL in special clinical scenarios

Certain obstetric conditions occur more commonly, therefore a brief overview of IOL in these conditions are highlighted.

9.1 Prolonged pregnancy

Prolonged pregnancy is a loose term that applies to all pregnancy beyond estimated due date which comprises of postdate and post term pregnancy. It occurs in about 5–10% of all pregnancy and the rate is reduced to incidence of 2–5% with ultrasound dating in the first trimester. A better classification of term pregnancy underscores the importance of late term (41 0/7–41 6/7 and post term (42 0/7 and beyond) on uteroplacental insufficiency with increase perinatal morbidity and mortality. The risk of still birth, macrosomia, shoulder dystocia, birth injury, postpartum haemorrhage and meconium aspiration syndrome are higher at late term and post term compared with early term (37 0/7–38 6/7) and full term (39 0/7–40 6/7) [13, 65]. Therefore, NICE guidelines and WHO recommends IOL at 41 weeks and beyond. In the rare circumstances when the woman declines IOL beyond 42 weeks, she should have twice weekly CTG and ultrasound and be counselled based on findings [1, 13]. Neonatal outcome did not improve following IOL at 39 weeks compared with expectant management in a multicenter trial (ARRIVE) in the United States, however the rate of caesarean section was lower in the intervention arm [66].

9.2 Hypertensive disorders of pregnancy

Hypertension complicates about 10% of pregnancies and remains one of the major causes of perinatal and maternal morbidity and mortality [67, 68]. Preeclampsia is considered a severe form of hypertension in pregnancy with an incidence of 2–5% of all hypertensions in pregnancy. Early onset (<34 weeks) and preterm preeclampsia (<37 weeks) could present with severe disease to prompt immediate delivery [68]. Following the HYPITAT Trial I, women with gestational hypertension or preeclampsia at term should be offered delivery. While HYPITAT II trial, recommends that non severe hypertension between 34 and 37 weeks should be delivered at 37 weeks [69, 70].

9.3 Prelabour rupture of membrane

The rupture of amniotic sac before the onset of labour is termed as prelabour rupture of membrane which can occur before (preterm prelabour rupture of membrane) or after 37 weeks of gestation (term prelabour rupture of membrane) [71]. Preterm (24/0–36/6) prelabour rupture of membrane (PPROM) complicates about 3% of pregnancies and is responsible for about 30–40% of preterm births. The Royal College of Obstetricians and Gynaecologists recommend conservative management for uncomplicated PPROM to 37 weeks. Prelabour rupture of membrane should be offered delivery after 37 weeks if it occurs and there is no onset of labour within 24 h or when PPROM is complicated by infection [72]. The induction method can either be by prostaglandin or oxytocin, however, the Bishop Score should be made favourable before such induction is embarked upon.

9.4 Hyperglycaemia in pregnancy

Hyperglycaemia is considered as one of the most common medical conditions in pregnancy with one in every 6 live births occurring in women with some degree of hyperglycaemia. Gestational Diabetes Mellitus is the most common type, and it is responsible for 84% of hyperglycaemia in pregnancy. There are higher incidences of perinatal and maternal morbidities and mortalities among pregnant women with any form of hyperglycaemia. A balance of glycaemic control and fetal maturity should be weighed to consider the timing of delivery. FIGO recommends delivery for women at 40–41 weeks for a well-controlled hyperglycaemia with fetal weight of <3800 g while delivery via induction is recommended at 38–39 weeks for poorly controlled hyperglycaemia with babies that are between 3800 and 4000 g. Elective caesarean section is the preferred delivery mode for babies weighing 4000 g and above [73].

9.5 IOL in previous caesarean section

The high rates of uterine rupture in patients with previous caesarean section is well established. There is a 2–3 times higher risk of uterine rupture in patient induced or augmented with previous caesarean section. This risk should be understood by both the physician preferably, a senior obstetrician, and the patient before undergoing induction or augmentation of labour in women with previous caesarean section. The risk of uterine rupture is lower with mechanical methods (Foley catheter and amniotomy) compared with prostaglandins [74].

10. Augmentation of labour (AOL)

Improving the efficiency of uterine contractions by increasing the frequency, duration, and intensity in women with inadequate or uncoordinated uterine contractions of spontaneous onset to reduce or prevent adverse outcome for the babies and their mother associated with prolonged labour is best describe as augmentation [75, 76]. The term AOL is loosely applied to women undergoing induction of labour, but this is a misnomer because contractions in induction of labour are not of spontaneous onset. The decision to augment the labour process should be carefully and meticulously evaluated after a thorough history and examination excluding any cephalopelvic disproportion and establishing that the cause of unsatisfactory progress of cervical dilatation and descent of the presenting part is solely the problems of power. Every local maternity setting should have a protocol of AOL using oxytocin infusion which is usually the same strength and frequency with induction protocol (see **Table 5**). Low dose oxytocin regimen is favoured because of less complications related to augmentation [76]. AROM can be considered as a sole method AOL because it enhances uterine contractions by increasing plasma prostaglandins, however the effectiveness of AROM appears to be debatable [77, 78].

Prior to preforming AROM, an informed consent is necessary, and patient should be informed of the benefits of AROM and the possible complications therein and the

Oxytocin regimens					
Time from start (min)	Oxytocin dose (mU/min)	Volume of infusion (ml/h)			
		10 IU in 500 ml	10 IU in 1000 ml	2 IU in 200 ml	10 IU in 1000 ml Without infusion set
0	1	3	6	6	10 drops
30	2	6	12	12	20 drops
60	4	12	24	24	30 drops
90	8	24	48	48	40 drops
120	12	36	72	72	50 drops
150	16	48	96	96	60 drops
180	20	60	120	120	
210	24	72	144	144	
240	28	84	168	168	
270	32	96	192	192	

Oxytocin dose of greater than 20 mU/min highlighted in red can only be administer by a specialist or a senior resident doctor.

Table 5.
Low dose oxytocin infusion for induction and augmentation of labour. Version (1.0) 2021.

fetal heart rate is checked. AROM can be performed with an Amniotomy finger cot (Amnicot) or Amniotomy hook (AmniHook) or a spinal needle for control release of amniotic fluid. The woman adopts a supine position and flexes her hips and knees (frog legged), or it can be done in the lithotomy position. A sterile glove finger is introduced using the dominant hand to performed vaginal examination and noting the cervical dilatation, effacement, position, station and to exclude cord presentation and possible vasa previa is noted. During the vaginal examination the amniotic perforator can be introduced with the non-dominant hand and the tip of the amniotomy hook is pushed against the sac with the index and middle finger guiding it and pull back. With successful rupture of membrane, the examining fingers should be held back to exclude cord prolapse and the amniotic fluid should be assessed for volume, colour, smell or particle within. It is good practice to recheck fetal heart and observe the woman closely for any vaginal bleeding [75, 76, 79]. For control release with spinal needle a bivalved speculum is required.

11. Complications of IOL and AOL

Artificial contractions are said to be more painful than spontaneous ones, more so the intensity and the duration might be more exaggerated than natural contractions. Therefore, the rates of complications associated with artificial uterine contractions are multiple folds compared with contractions from spontaneous onset [13]. The complications of IOL and AOL could range from tachysystole, hypertonus or an outright tachysystole with fetal heart rate abnormalities, placenta abruption or uterine rupture [80, 81] which occur in about 1–5% of women undergoing IOL. It is estimated that

IOL could fail in 15% of patient with unfavourable cervix [81]. Both IOL and AOL could result in cord prolapse following AROM. There is a tendency of increasing the risk of infection, operative vaginal delivery and increased caesarean section rate [80] in women undergoing IOL. Poor childbirth experience was encountered in about 4.5% of patient undergoing IOL in a recent study to assess maternal childbirth experience [82]. The risk of primary post-partum haemorrhage in patients undergoing IOL is well documented [83]. Fetal complications can be in the form of fetal distress, meconium stained liquor and neonatal jaundice. Litigation from the abuse of oxytocin has been enormous in the past decade globally [84].

12. Conclusion

There is an increased rate of IOL especially across developed countries, however the unmet need for IOL in developing countries is bridged by the availability of misoprostol and Foley's catheter at cost effective rates. Timely and appropriate IOL can lead to reduction in perinatal and maternal morbidity and mortality. Therefore, there is need for obstetricians and physicians that provide care in women's health to keep abreast with the best external available evidence on the subject matter. It is important to employ the concept of respectful maternity in the pre-induction, induction, and post induction phase to improve outcomes, reduce litigations and enhance women satisfaction. A diagnosis of failed induction does not translate to automatic caesarean section if the fetal and maternal conditions are adjudged to be normal and stable; a pause and restart can be initiated after 24–48 h with lower threshold for intervention in the second cycle.

Author details

Benjamin Joseph Nggada
Department of Maternal and Child Health, University of Namibia, Windhoek, Namibia

*Address all correspondence to: bilyaminu@hotmail.com

References

[1] World Health Organization (WHO). Recommendations: Induction of Labour at or Beyond Term. Geneva: World Health Organization; 2018 http://apps.who.int/iris/bitstream/handle/10665/44531/9789241501156_eng.pdf?sequence=1

[2] Marconi AM. Recent advances in the induction of labor. F1000Research. 2019;**8**(F1000 Faculty Rev):1829. DOI: 10.12688/f1000research.17587.1

[3] World Health Organization (WHO). Recommendations: Intrapartum Care for a Positive Childbirth Experience. Geneva: World Health Organization; 2018 Licence: CC BY-NC-SA 3.0 IGO

[4] Akuamoah-Boateng J, Spencer R. Woman-centered care: Women's experiences and perceptions of induction of labor for uncomplicated post-term pregnancy: A systematic review of qualitative evidence. Midwifery. 2018; **67**:46-56. DOI: 10.1016/j.midw.2018.08.018 Epub 5 September 2018. PMID: 30232052

[5] Gomez HB, Hoffman MK, Caplan R, Ruhsta K, Young MHH, Sciscione DOAC. Buccal vs vaginal misoprostol combined with Foley catheter for cervical ripening at term (the BIGIN trial): A randomized controlled trial. American Journal of Obstetrics and Gynecology. 2021; **224**(524):e1-e8

[6] National Health Service. Rise in proportion of induced labours, new maternity figure shows. 2018. NHS Maternity statistics 2017-2018. Published on 25 October 2081 by NHS Digital. https://digital.nhs.uk/news/2018/nhs-maternity-statistics-2017-18

[7] Carter S, Channon A, Berrington. Socioeconomic risk factors for labour induction in the United Kingdom. BMC Pregnancy and Childbirth. 2020; **20**(146). DOI: 10.1186/s12884-020-2840-3

[8] Wilson BL. Assessing the effects of age, gestation, socioeconomic status, and ethnicity on labor inductions. Journal of Nursing Scholarship. 2007;**39**:208-213

[9] Rydahl E, Declercq E, Juhl M, Maimburg RD. Routine induction in late-term pregnancies: follow-up of a Danish induction of labour paradigm. BMJ Open. 2019;**9**:e032815. DOI: 10.1136/bmjopen-2019-032815 https://bmjopen.bmj.com/content/9/12/e032815

[10] Lueth GD, Kebede A, Medhanyie AA. Prevalence, outcomes and associated factors of labour induction among women delivered at public hospitals at MEKELLE town-(a hospital based cross sectional study). BMC Pregnancy and Childbirth. 2020; **20**:203. DOI: 10.1186/s12884-020-02862-7

[11] Vogel JP, Souza JP, Gulmezoglu AM. Patterns and outcomes of induction of labour in Africa and Asia: A secondary analysis of the WHO global survey on maternal and neonatal health. PLoS One. 2013;**8**(6):11. https://journals.plos.org/plosone/article/file?id=10.1371/journal.pone.0065612&type=printable

[12] Society of Obstetrician and Gynaecology of Canada (SOGC). Induction of labour. SOGC Clinical Practice Guideline. No 296. Journal of Obstetrics and Gynaecology Canada. 2013;**35**(9):840-857

[13] National Institute for Health and Care Excellence (NICE). Inducing Labour. 2021. www.nice.org.uk/guidance/ng207

[14] Melkie A, Addisu D, Mekie M, Dagnew E. Failed inductionmof labour and its associated factors in Ethopia: A systematic review and metaanlysis. Heilyon. 2021;**7**(3):e06415. https://www.cell.com/heliyon/pdf/S2405-8440(21)00520-X.pdf

[15] Banos N, Migliorelli F, Posadas E, Ferreri J, Palacio M. Definition of failed induction of labour and its predictive factors: Two unsolved issues of everyday clinical situation. Fetal Diagnosis and Therapy. 2015;**38**:161-169. DOI: 10.1159/000433429

[16] Pierce S, Bakker R, Myers DA, Edwards RK. Clinical insight for cervical ripening and labour induction using prostaglandins. The American Journal of Perinatology. 2018;**8**:e307-e314

[17] Macones GA, Hankins GD, Spong CY, Hauth J, Moore T. The 2008 National Institute of Child Health and Human Development workshop report on electronic fetal monitoring: Update on definitions, interpretation, and research guidelines. Obstetrics and Gynecology. 2008;**112**:661-666

[18] Sukumaran S, Jia YJ, Chandraharan E. Uterine tachysystole, hypertonus and hyperstimulation: An urgent need to get the definitions right to avoid intrapartum hypoxic-ischaemic brain injury. Global Journal of Reproductive Medicine. 2021;**8**(2):5556735. DOI: 10.19080/GJORM.2021.08.5556735

[19] Mealing NM, Roberts CL, Ford JB, Simpson JM, Morris JM. Trends in induction of labour, 1998–2007: A population-based study. The Australian and New Zealand Journal of Obstetrics and Gynaecology. 2009;**49**:599-605

[20] Nguyen-Ngo C, Lappas M. Mechanism of normal labour. Current Opinion in Physiology. 2020;**13**:27-32. DOI: 10.1016/j.cophys.2019.09.008

[21] Nadeem L, Shynlova O, Matysiak-Zablocki E, Mesiano S, Dong X, Lye S. Molecular evidence of functional progesterone withdrawal in human myometrium. Nature Communications. 2016;**7**:11565. DOI: 10.1038/ncomms11565

[22] Nadeem L, Shynlova O, Mesiano S, Lye S. Progesterone via its type-A receptor promotes myometrial gap junction coupling. Scientific Reports. 2017;**7**:13357. DOI: 10.1038/s41598-017-13488-9

[23] Shmigol AV, Eisner DA, Wray S. Simultaneous measurements of changes in sarcoplasmic reticulum and cytosolic. The Journal of Physiology. 2001;**531**:707-713. DOI: 10.1111/j.1469-7793.2001.0707h.x

[24] New Zealand College of Midwives. Helping Women Make Decisions about Induction of Labour. https://www.midwife.org.nz/wp-content/uploads/2020/01/ARRIVE-Infographic-amended.pdf.

[25] The Federation of Obstetricians and Gynaecologist of India, Indian College of Obstetrician and Gynaecologist (FOGSI-ICOG). Induction of Labour: Good Clinical Practice Recommendation. 2018. https://www.fogsi.org/wp-content/uploads/2018/09/XGCPR-IOL-26July.pdf.

[26] Bishop EH. Pelvic scoring for elective induction of elective induction. Obstetrics and Gynecology. 1988;**24**:266-268

[27] Leppert PC. Anatomy and physiology of cervical ripening. Clinical Obstetrics and Gynecology. 1995;**38**(2):267-279. DOI: 10.1097/00003081-199506000-00009 PMID: 7554594

[28] Schmitz T, Fuchs F, Closset E, et al. Outpatient cervical ripening by nitric oxide donors for prolonged pregnancy: A randomized controlled trial. Obstetrics and Gynecology. 2014;**124**(6):1089-1097

[29] Promsonthi P, Preechapornprasert D, Chanrachakul B. Nitric oxide donors for cervical ripening in first-trimester surgical abortion. Cochrane Database Syst Rev. 2011;7(12):CD007444. DOI: 10.1002/14651858.CD007444.pub3

[30] Bishop EH. Pelvic Scoring for Elective Induction. International Journal of Gynecology & Obstetrics. 1964;**24**: 266-8

[31] Calder AA, Embrey MP, Hillier K. Extra-amniotic prostaglandin E2 for induction of labour at term. The Journal of Obstetrics and Gynaecology of the British Commonwealth. 1974;**81**:39-46

[32] Galzie SK, Rao SB. Cervical effacement, as an independent parameter versus modified bishop score, for predicting the favourability of vaginal delivery in a primigravida at 40 weeks of gestation and beyond. Iternational Journal of Reproduction, Contraception, Obstetrics and Gynecology. 2020;**9**(5):1-7

[33] Ikeotuonye AC, Anikwe CC, Obuna JA, Okorochukwu BC, Eijkeme BN, Ifemelumma CC, et al. Relationship between Bishop score and success of induction of labour in Federal Teaching Hospital, Abakaliki, Ebonyi state. Open Journal of Obstetrics and Gynecology. 2018;**8**:980-992. DOI: 10.4236/ojog.2018.811099

[34] Kehila M, Bougmiza I, Ben Hmid R, Abdelfatteh W, Mahjoub S, Channoufi MB. Bishop score vs ultrasound cervical length in the preinduction of cervical ripening success and vaginal delivery in nulliparous women. Minerva Ginecologica. 2015; **67**(6):499-505

[35] American College of Obstetricians and Gynaecologists (ACOG). ACOG Patient Safety Checklist No 2. Inpatient Induction of Labor Committee Opinion, No.560, 2013; December 2011, reaffirmed 2014, Available from: https://obgynriskalliance.com/globalassets/ob-gyn-tool-kit/acog-patient-safety-checklists/acog-patient-safety-checklist-inpatient-induction-of-labor.pdf

[36] Thomas J, Fairclough A, Kavanagh J, Kelly AJ. Vaginal prostaglandin (PGE2 and PGF2a) for induction of labour at term. Cochrane Database of Systematic Reviews. 2014;**6**:CD003101

[37] Kwawukume EY, Ayertey RP. Misoprostol for induction of labour in a low-resource setting. Tropical Journal of Obstetrics and Gynaecology. 2002;**19**(2): 78-81

[38] Helmig RB, Hildman LE. An audit of oral administration of Angusta® (misoprostol) 25 μg for induction of labor in 976 consecutive women with a singleton pregnancy in a university hospital in Denmark. Acta Obstetricia et Gynecologica Scandinavica. 2020;**99**: 1396-1402

[39] DebBarma AM, Baidya JL, Ray D. A comparative study of misoprostol oral versus vaginal route for induction of labour. International Journal of Reproduction, Contraception, Obstetrics and Gynecology. 2020;**9**(5): 1907-1913

[40] Tseng J-Y, Lin I-C, Chang W-H, Yeh C-C, Horng H-C, Wang PH. Using dinoprostone vaginal insert for induction of labor: A single institute experience. Taiwanese Journal of Obstetrics & Gynecology. 2020;**59**:723-727

[41] Reinhard J, Rosler R, Yuan J, Schiermeier S, Herrmann E, Eichbaum MH, et al. Prostaglandin E2 labour induction with intravaginal (Minprostin) versus intracervical (Prepidil) administration at term: Randomized study of maternal and neonatal outcome and patient's perception using the Osgood semantic differential scales. BioMed Research International. 2014;**2014**:682919. DOI: 10.1155/2014/682919

[42] Morris JL, Winikoff B, Dabash R, Weeks A, Faundes A, Gemzell-Danielson K, et al. FIGO updated recommendation for misoprostol used alone in gynecology and obstetrics. International Journal of Gynecology & Obstetrics. 2017;**138**: 363-366

[43] Baranowska B, Kajdy A, Kiersnowska I, et al. Oxytocin administration for induction and augmentation of labour in polish maternity units—An observational study. BMC Pregnancy and Childbirth. 2021:**21**: 764. DOI: 10.1186/s12884-021-04190-w

[44] Kenyon S, Tokumasu H, Dowswell T, Pledge D, Mori R. High-dose versus low-dose oxytocin for augmentation of delayed labour. Cochrane pregnancy and childbirth group, editor. Cochrane Database of Systematic Reviews [Internet]. 2013;**13** [cited 13 February 2021]; Available from: http://dpo.wiley.com/10.1002/14651858.CD007201.pub3

[45] Ferguson JE II, Head BH, Frank FH, Singer JS, Stefos T, Mari G. Misoprostol versus low-dose oxytocin for cervical ripening: A prospective, randomized, double-mask trial. American Journal of Obstetrics and Gynecology. 2002;**187**(2): 273-280

[46] Esakoff TF, Kilpatrick SJ. The transcervical foley balloon. Contemporary obstetrics and gynaecology. 2013. https://www.contemporaryobgyn.net/view/transcervical-foley-balloon

[47] Liu X, Wang Y, Zhang F, et al. Double-versus single-balloon catheters for labour induction and cervical ripening: A meta-analysis. BMC Pregnancy and Childbirth. 2019;**19**:358. DOI: 10.1186/s12884-019-2491-4

[48] Jozwiak M, Bloemenkamp KW, Kelly AJ, Mol BW, Irion O, Boulvain M. Mechanical methods for induction of labour. The Cochrane Database of Systematic Reviews. 2012;**14**(3): CD001233. DOI: 10.1002/14651858.CD001233.pub2. PMID: 22419277

[49] Levy R, Kanengiser B, Furman B, Arie AB, Brown D, Hagay ZJ. A randomized trial comparing a 30 ml and an 80 ml Foley catheter balloon for preinduction cervical ripening. American Journal of Obstetrics and Gynecology. 2004;**191**(5):1632-1636

[50] Cherian AG, Marcus TA, Sebastine T, Rathore S, Mathews JE. Induction of labour using Foley catheter with weight attached versus without weight attached: A randomized control trial. The International Journal of Gynecology. 2022;**157**(1):159-164

[51] Pennell CE, Henderson JJ, O'Neill MJ, McChlery S, Doherty DA, Dickinson JE. Induction of labour in nulliparous women with an unfavourable cervix; a randomized controlled trial comparing double and single balloon catheters and PGE2 gel. BJOG : An International Journal of Obstetrics and Gynaecology. 2009;**116**(11): 1443-1452

[52] Sciscione AC, Muench M, Pollock M, Jenkins TM, Tildon-Burton J, Colmorgen GHC. Transcervical Foley catheter for preinduction cervical

ripening in an outpatient versus inpatient setting. Obstetrics and Gynecology. 2001;**98**(5.1):751-756

[53] Sullivan CA, Benton LW, Roach H, Smith LG Jr, Martin RW, Morrison JC. Combining medical and mechanical methods of cervical ripening. Does it increase the likelihood of successful induction of labor? The Journal of Reproductive Medicine. 1996;**41**(11): 823-828

[54] Dalui R, Suri V, Ray P, Gupta I. Comparison of extraamniotic Foley catheter and intracervical prostaglandin E gel for preinduction cervical ripening. Acta Obstetricia et Gynecologica Scandinavica. 2005;**84**(4):362-367

[55] Moraes Filho OB, Albuquerque RM, Cecatti JG. A randomized controlled trial comparing vaginal misoprostol versus Foley catheter plus oxytocin for labor induction. Acta Obstetricia et Gynecologica Scandinavica. 2010;**89**(8): 1045-1052

[56] Gomez HB, Hoffman MK, Caplan R, Ruhstaller K, Young MHH, Sciscione AC. Buccal vs vaginal misoprostol combined with Foley catheter for cervical ripening at term: A randomized controlled trial. American Journal of Obstetrics and Gynecology. 2021;**224**(524):e1-e8

[57] Sukumaran S, Chandraharan E. The historical practice of "membrane sweep" to initiate labour: Does it have a role in contemporary obstetric practice? Global Journal of Reproductive Medicine. 2021; **8**(2):5556733. DOI: 10.19080/GJORM.2021.08.5556733

[58] Finucane EM, Murphy DJ, Biesty LM, Gyte GML, Cotter AM, et al. Membrane sweeping for induction of6labour. Cochrane Database of Systematic Reviews. 2020;**2**(1): CD000451

[59] Yaddehige SS, Kalansooriya HD, Rameez MFM. Comparison of cervical massage with membrane sweeping for pre-induction cervical ripening at term: A randomized control trial. Sri Lanka Journal of Obstetrics and Gynaecology. 2019;**41**:66-74. DOI: 10.4038/sljog.v41i3.7883

[60] Jeeva MA, Dommisse J. Laminaria tents or vaginal prostaglandins for cervical ripening: A comparative trial. South African Medical Journal. 1982;**61**: 402-403

[61] Chodankar R, Sood A, Gupta J. An overview of the past, current and future trends for cervical ripening in induction of labour. The Obstetrician and Gynaecologist. 2017;**19**:219-226. DOI: 10.1111/tog.12395

[62] ClinicalTrials.gov. Dilapan-S/Dilasoft E-Registry in Induction of Labor (DSREGISTRYIL) https://clinicaltrials.gov/ct2/show/NCT02318173

[63] Tan PC, Soe MZ, Sulaiman S, Omar SZ. Immediate compared with delayed oxytocin after amniotomy labor induction in parous women: A randomized controlled trial. Obstetrics and Gynecology. 2013;**121**:253-259

[64] Mozurkewich EL, Chilimigras JL, Berman DR, Perni UC, Romero VC, Valerie JK, et al. Methods of induction of labour: A systematic review. BMC Pregnancy and Childbirth. 2011;**11**:84 http://www.biomedcentral.com/1471-2393/11/84

[65] Hellmeyer L, Bahlman F, Janku P, Zahumensky J, Baev O, Saad A, Murthy A. ClinicalTrials.gov. Dilapan-S/Dilasoft E-Registry in Induction of Labor (DSREGISTRYIL). https://clinicaltrials.gov/ct2/show/NCT02318173

[66] Grobman WA, Rice MM, Reddy UM, Tita AT, Silver RM, Mallett G, et al. Labor induction versus expectant management in low-risk nulliparous women. The New England Journal of Medicine. 2018;**379**: 513-523

[67] National Institute for Health and Care Excellence (NICE). Hypertension in pregnancy: diagnosis and management. NICE guideline [NG133]. 2019 www.nice.org.uk/guidance/ng133

[68] Poon LC, Shennan A, Hyett JA, Kapur A. Hadar E, Divakar H et al. The International Federation of Gynecology and Obstetrics (FIGO) initiative on pre-eclampsia: A pragmatic guide for first-trimester screening and prevention. International Journal of Gynaecology and Obstetrics. 2019;**145**(Suppl. 1):1-33

[69] Koopmans CM, Bijlenga D, Groen H, MC Vijgen S, Aarnoudse JG, Bekedem DJ et al. HYPITAT study group. Induction of labour versus expectant monitoring for gestational hypertension or mild pre-eclampsia after 36 weeks' gestation (HYPITAT): A multicentre, open-label randomised controlled trial. Lancet 2009;**374**(9694):979-988

[70] Broekhuijsen K, van Baaren G-J, van Pampus MG, Ganzevoort W, Sikkema JM, Woiski M, et al. Immediate delivery versus expectant monitoring for hypertensive disorders of pregnancy between 34 and 37 weeks of gestation (HYPITAT II): An open -label, randomized controlled trial. Lancet. 2015;**385**(9986):2492-2501

[71] Tiruye G, Shiferaw K, Tura AK, Debella A, Musa A. Prevalence of premature rupture of membrane and its associated factors among pregnant women in Ethiopia: A systematic review and meta-analysis. SAGE Open Medicine. 2021;**9**:1-9

[72] Thomson AJ, On behalf of the Royal College of Obstetricians and Gynaecologists. Care of Women Presenting with suspected preterm prelabour rupture of membranes from 24+0 weeks of gestation. BJOG. 2019; **126**:e152-e166

[73] Hod M, Kapur A, Sacks DA, Hadar E, Agarwal M, Di Renzo GC. The International Federation of Gynecology and Obstetrics (FIGO) initiative on gestational diabetes mellitus: A pragmatic guide for diagnosis, management, and care. International Journal of Gynecology & Obstetrics. 2015;**131**:S173-S211

[74] Royal College of Obstetricians and Gynaecologists. Green-top guideline No. 45 Birth after previous caesarean section. October 2015 London: RCOG; Available at: www.rcog.org.uk

[75] Nabhan A, Boulvain M. Augmentation of labour. Best Practice. 2020;**67**:80-89

[76] World Health Organization (WHO). WHO recommendation for augmentation of labour. 2014. https://apps.who.int/iris/bitstream/10665/112825/1/9789241507363_eng.pdf

[77] Mitchell MD, Flint AP, Bibby J, Brunt J, Arnold JM, Anderson AB. Rapid increases in plasma prostaglandin concentrations after vaginal examination and amniotomy. British Medical Journal. 1977;**2**(6096):1183-1185

[78] Wei S, Wo BL, Qi HP, Xu H, Luo ZC, Roy C, Fraser WD. Early amniotomy and early oxytocin for prevention of, or therapy for, delay in first stage spontaneous labour compared with routine care. Cochrane Database Syst Rev. 2012;**9**(9):CD006794. DOI: 10.1002/14651858.CD006794.pub3

[79] Mahdy H, Glowacki C, Eruo FU. Amniotomy. [Updated 25 August 2021]. In: StatPearls [Internet]. Treasure Island (FL): StatPearls Publishing; 2022 Available from: https://www.ncbi.nlm.nih.gov/books/NBK470167/

[80] Devarasetty S, Habeebullah S. Induction of labor: A review. Journal of Basic, Clinical and Applied Health Science. 2019;**2**(4):128-133

[81] National Collaborating Centre for Women's and Children's Health (UK). Induction of Labour. London: RCOG Press; 2008. https://pubmed.ncbi.nlm.nih.gov/21510026/ PMID: 21510026

[82] Adler K, Rahkonen L, Kruit H. Maternal childbirth experience in induced and spontaneous labour measured in a visual analog scale and the factors influencing it; a two-year cohort study. BMC Pregnancy and Childbirth. 2020;**20**:415. DOI: 10.1186/s12884-020-03106-4

[83] Kumar B, Kumari S, Hughes S, Savill S. Prospective cohort study of induction of labor: Indications, outcome and postpartum hemorrhage. The European Journal of Midwifery. 2021;**5**: 53. DOI: 10.18332/ejm/142782

[84] Olah KDJ, Steer P. The use and abuse of oxytocin. Obstetrics and Gynecology. 2015;**17**:265-271

Section 3

Delivery

Chapter 4

Update and Trend in Episiotomy Practice

Francis Pebolo Pebalo and Jackline Ayikoru

Abstract

Episiotomy is one of the most commonly practiced obstetric procedures done to enlarge the diameter of the vulval outlet to facilitate the passage for the fetal head and prevent an uncontrolled tear of the perineal tissues in the second stage of labor. Historically, the procedure was indicated to prevent third- or fourth-degree perineal tears as well as for prolonged second stage, macrosomia, non-reassuring fetal heart rate, instrumental delivery, occiput posterior position, and shoulder dystocia. Routine episiotomy is now considered to be obstetrics violence, rates of not exceeding 10% have been recommended by World Health Organization (WHO). Despite this recommendation, episiotomy is still practiced routinely in many settings.

Keywords: episiotomy, obstetric anal sphincter injuries (OASIs), redness, ecchymosis, edema, discharge and apposition (REEDA), scale restrictive episiotomy, and mediolateral episiotomy

1. Introduction

Episiotomy is a surgical cut in the tissue between the vagina and the anus (called the perineum) made just before delivery. It is one of the most commonly practiced obstetric procedures done to enlarge the diameter of the vulval outlet to facilitate the passage for the fetal head and prevent an uncontrolled tear of the perineal tissues in the second stage of labor [1–3]. The procedure was introduced into obstetric practice without any sound scientific evidence corroborating any possible benefits [4]. It was promoted in the twentieth century by renowned interventionists, obstetricians such as Gabe and De Lee [5]. Their perception was that the female body was essentially defective and dependent on medical interventions to enable childbirth [5]. In 1970s, there was disagreement in the practice especially because of pressure from the women's movements demanding changes in the obstetric model [4].

In 1983, Thacker and Banta gave a full account of the lack of scientific data supporting the use of episiotomy and the potential danger associated with the procedure [3]. Historical indications such as a prolonged second stage, macrosomia, non-reassuring fetal heart rate, instrumental delivery, occiput posterior position, and shoulder dystocia have been questioned [6].

Routine episiotomy is now considered to be obstetrics violence when a woman is automatically transformed into a patient and when routine medical procedures are carried out without giving the woman the right to make her own decisions concerning her own body [7].

1.1 Types of episiotomy

The most commonly practiced and accepted type of episiotomy is the mediolateral, owing to its protective roles in preventing obstetric anal sphincter injury (OASI) [8]. Median/midline episiotomy, although has a bigger risk of causing OASI, is praised for causing less pain/bleeding, ease in repair, and healing more easily [9]. A clear illustration and description of the type of episiotomy can be seen in **Figure 1** and **Table 1**. Other reported episiotomy types in literature are lateral episiotomy, which was condemned, and also a J-shaped episiotomy incision that is not commonly practiced.

Figure 1 has been adopted and modified from [10].

1.2 Episiotomy repair

Episiotomy incision is generally repaired after delivery of placenta to achieve hemostasis and approximate lacerated tissues. The aseptic procedure is carried out in a well-lit room with adequate exposure and appropriate instruments and anesthesia. Since most if not all repairs are done in laboring wards, adequate local or regional analgesia is used. Extension to a third- or fourth-degree perineal tear may necessitate examination under anesthesia and requires regional or general anesthesia that is done in an operating theater.

A suture is placed approximately a centimeter proximal to the apex of the incision within the vagina and secured with a knot, vaginal mucosa, and sub-mucosa are sutured up to the hymeneal ring, perineal muscles are then approximated followed by the closure of perineal skin using a continuous subcutaneous suturing technique [11]. Continuous stitching technique is preferred to interrupted as it is associated with less pain, easily performed by the inexperienced operator, and economical [12].

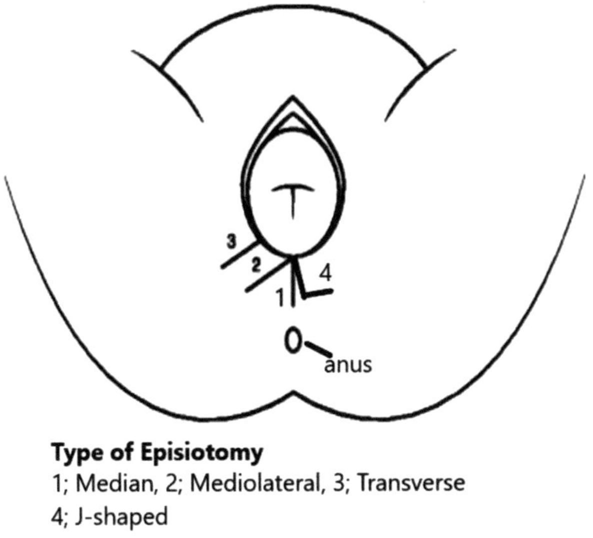

Figure 1.
Illustration of episiotomy types.

Type of episiotomy	
Definition	**Way of execution**
Median	The incision starts at the posterior fourchette and runs along the midline through the center of the perineal body. The incision should run for approximately half of the length of the perineum (2–3 cm) without affecting the anal muscle
Mediolateral	An incision is performed downward and outward from the midpoint of the fourchette, either to the right or left toward the ischial tuberosity with 3–4 cm length, beginning in the midline and directed laterally, and downward away from the rectum. It affects the skin, subcutaneous tissue, bulbospongiosus muscle, superficial transverse perineal muscle, and the levator
Lateral	The incision starts from about 1 cm (0.4 in) away from the center of the fourchette and extends laterally. Possible complications comprise injury to the Bartholin's duct, which is why lateral incisions are deemed inadvisable by most specialists and rarely mentioned in the obstetric literature
J-shaped episiotomy	It entails a midline incision, curved laterally away from the anus. Curved scissors are used starting in the midline of the vagina until the incision is 2·5° cm from the anus, then directing the incision toward the ischial tuberosity away from the anal sphincter
Radical lateral (Schuchardt incision)	Generally considered a non-obstetrical incision, it is a fully extended episiotomy, deep into one vaginal sulcus and is curved downward and laterally partway around the rectum. It may be carried out at the beginning of radical vaginal hysterectomy or trachelectomy to allow easy access to the parametrium, to enable extraction of a neglected vaginal pessary, or quite rarely, to facilitate childbirth if complications arise (fetal macrosomia, difficult breech, or shoulder dystocia)

Adopted from [9].

Table 1.
Type of episiotomy.

1.3 Current trend in episiotomy practice

Episiotomy is practiced in varied ways with differing prevalence ranging from as low as less than 1/3 to as high as 86% [13] depending on whether it is used routinely or in a restricted way.

World Health Organization (WHO) Guideline Developing Groups emphasized the need for health systems to adopt a policy of restrictive rate of not more than 10% rather than routine use of episiotomy to reduce its potential complications and the use of additional resources for its treatment [14] as restrictive episiotomy has shown benefits [15]. Restrictive other than routine episiotomy protocol has been supported by FIGO [16], a mediolateral episiotomy type is the one recommended, and this should be performed under adequate analgesia, whether anesthesia is already in place for labor, such as epidural, or by administering a local infiltration [16].

Despite the controversy regarding the validity of episiotomy's routine use in obstetrics and the fact that liberal use of the procedure has been discouraged, this is still one of the most commonly performed obstetric procedures worldwide [17, 18]. Although this restrictive episiotomy practice has shown many benefits, especially regarding the reduction of injuries to the posterior perineum, the strictest definition of restrictive use was to avoid episiotomy unless indicated for fetal well-being. Other definitions of restrictive episiotomy are to "avoid the procedure," use only when "medically necessary," or not perform an episiotomy to avoid a laceration [19]. The balance between risk and benefit for episiotomy is therefore not entirely straightforward. An episiotomy may be unavoidable if the baby needs to be delivered quickly.

The lack of evidence supporting episiotomy benefits has caused a significant decline in the practice in most countries. In France, a decline from 15.5% in 2013 to 9.3% in 2017 has been realized [20], and for operative vaginal births, there had been a varied decrease in episiotomy rates from as low as 25% to as high as 75% in some geographical location in France [21].

1.4 Indications

Historical indications for episiotomy included: abnormal progress of labor, non-reassuring fetal status, prematurity, assisted vaginal delivery, shoulder dystocia. It was also believed to hasten the second stage of labor, decrease pelvic floor disorder and sexual dysfunction, reduce urinary and fecal incontinence [15]. Several guidelines recommend the use of mediolateral episiotomy for the prevention of obstetric anal sphincter injuries (OASI) [8]. Episiotomy plays the main role during assisted vaginal birth as this is related to the increased incidence of OASI. The procedure can be indicated when there is a high likelihood of third-degree or fourth-degree perineal tear, soft tissue dystocia, a requirement to accelerate delivery of a compromised fetus, and need to facilitate operative vaginal delivery or a history of female genital mutilation [22].

1.5 Factors associated with episiotomy

Varied risk and protective factors are influencing the practice of episiotomy in obstetrics. The risk factors include primiparity [23, 24], absence of prior vaginal birth, assisted vaginal delivery are among the predictive factors influencing episiotomy practice. In some settings, episiotomy operations were being performed to allow midwifery and medical students the opportunity to learn and practice the procedure [24]. Being an adolescent and having other medical conditions while pregnant is associated with the procedure [25].

Factors that are protective against episiotomy include perineal massage. This procedure can be done especially in the second stage of labor [26–28]. The procedure is an effective approach to increasing the chance of delivery with intact perineum especially for women with a first vaginal birth [29]. In other literature, massage can be started as early as 34 weeks of gestation, and it is done with oil for 5–10 min every day to increase flexibility and elasticity [30]. In addition to massage, perineal support and warm compresses during the second stage are protective for episiotomy and anal sphincter injury [30].

Another important innovative tool to reduce the risk of episiotomy is an Epi-No device, developed in early 2000, to facilitate a natural birth and reduce the risk of perineal injury including needs for episiotomy. The Epi-No device is promising, with potentially positive effects on a natural birth without major complications [31].

1.6 Obstetric anal sphincter injuries (OASI)

OASI are injuries that involve the anal sphincter. It is dreaded complication after a vaginal delivery that has significant maternal morbidity such as perineal pain, dyspareunia, flatulence, and anal incontinence [32].

OASI either involves third or fourth-degree perineal tears. A third-degree perineal tear is defined as a partial or complete disruption of the anal sphincter muscles, a fourth-degree involves the rectal mucosa [33] as seen in **Table 2** and **Figure 2**.

Third-degree tear	**Injury to the perineum involving the anal sphincter complex**
3A	Less than 50% of EAS thickness torn
3B	More than 50% of EAS thickness torn
3C	Both EAS and IAS torn
Fourth-degree tear	Injury to perineum involving the anal sphincter complex (both EAS and IAS) and anal epithelium
Buttonhole tear	External anal sphincter intact but anal or rectal mucosa with or without internal anal sphincter tear

Adopted from [34].
Key: IAS, internal anal sphincter; EAS, external anal sphincter.

Table 2.
Description of OASI.

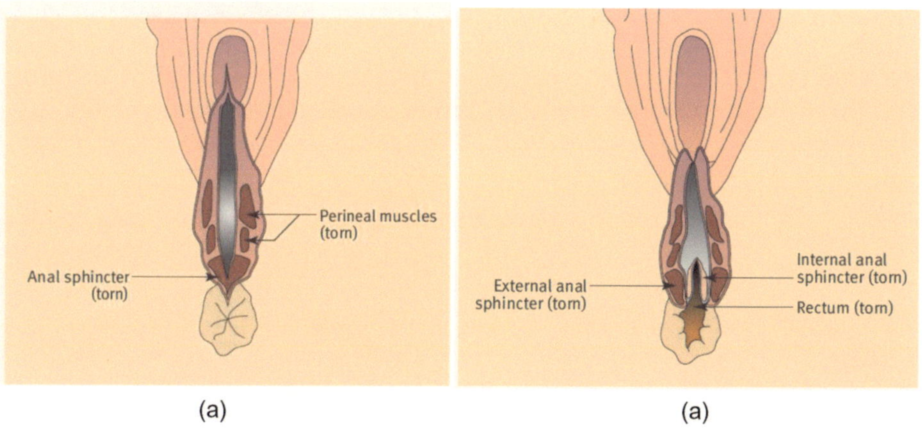

Figure 2.
OASI; (a) third-degree perineal tear, (b) fourth-degree perineal tear. Adopted from [35].

The risk of getting OASI can be done by relieving pressure on the central posterior perineum by an episiotomy and/or controlled delivery of the head. An episiotomy aimed at 60° from the midline has been seen to be protective for OASI [36]; hence, the introduction of episiotomy scissors specially designed to achieve a cutting angle of 60°, EPISCISSORS-60® [37]. Vacuum-assisted delivery and bigger babies were seen to be an important independent factor in one cohort study [38].

1.6.1 OASI repair—sphincteroplasty

A repair can be done primarily if OASI is diagnosed following vaginal delivery, and this represents the mainstay of treatment. A delay of up to 12 h is allowable if resources for repair are not available. A secondary repair can be done later when tissue edema has subsided for cases diagnosed later or if injuries have been unrepaired for more than 12 h, and this is referred to as secondary repair [39].

The aim of sphincter repair (either primary or secondary) is to restore a functioning anal canal by reconstruction of a muscular cylinder that is at least 2 cm thick and 3 cm long [39].

Meticulous hemostasis and anatomic approximation with a multilayer closure of all disrupted tissue layers are the key principles for preventing complications and restoring fecal continence and two recognized methods for the repair of OASI: end-to-end (approximation) and overlap repair [39] are important depending on the extent of the injuries as illustrated in **Figure 3**.

An overlap is more superior to an end-to-end method in terms of reduction in perineal pain, dyspareunia, flatus incontinence, and fecal incontinence [39, 40].

Although the repair techniques have been well documented, the confidence in detecting OASI and competence in the repair of OASI does not correlate with knowledge of anatomy and risk factors of OASI in a survey among obstetricians [41].

1.7 Complications

The suitability of routine use of episiotomy has been questioned by specialists and scientific societies, and several professional medical associations and patient and women's rights advocates have been associating it with obstetric violence [9]. Episiotomy has been associated with the risk of repeat episiotomy in the subsequent birth due to tighter perineum and weaker scar [42]. Post episiotomy pain is common after delivery, and this may end up in pain at first intercourse especially if it occurs in the first 3 months after delivery [43]. The risk is higher if intercourse occurs within the first 6 weeks after delivery and in some cases, women present with gaping

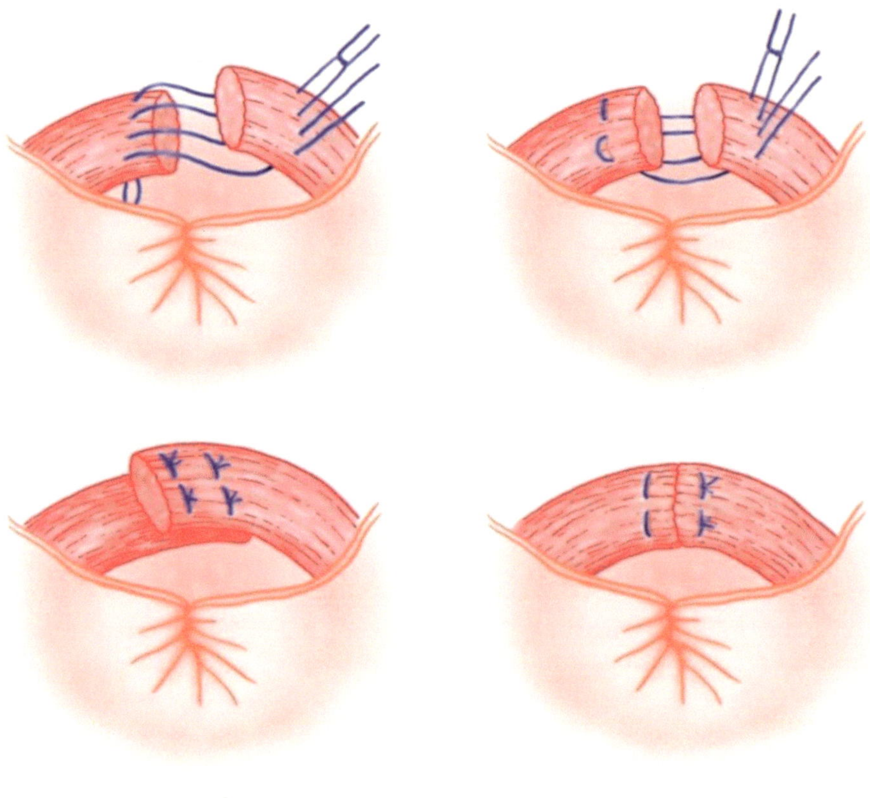

Figure 3.
Episiotomy repair technique. Adopted from [39].

episiotomy wounds following intercourse [44]. The incision substantially increases maternal blood loss, the average depth of posterior perineal injury, risk of anal sphincter damage, improper wound healing, increased amount of pain in the first several postpartum days, and infection [45]. Episiotomy at the first vaginal birth significantly and independently increases the risk of repeated episiotomy and spontaneous tears in subsequent delivery [42, 46].

Episiotomy-related morbidity can be measured using the Redness, Ecchymosis, Edema, Discharge, and Apposition scale (REEDA scale) [47]. Higher REEDA scores denote poor healing process or severe trauma to the perineal tissue as shown in one of our studies in Mulago Hospital in Uganda [48]. The rate of the gaping wound is particularly higher among those done episiotomy compared with spontaneous perineal tear [48], and this can be attributed to the fact that spontaneous perineal tear occurs normally along the natural tissue planes, and it's easier to repair compared with episiotomy. A similar study in Mulago relates episiotomy to increased risk of infection and the need for secondary re-suturing [49].

Episiotomy-related pain has been shown to persist for more than 14 days after delivery [48] supporting claims that cutting across tissue planes is associated with more pain compared with spontaneous tear that normally follows the natural tissue planes as reported by [3, 50, 51] and that episiotomy is a painful policy [2]. A meta-analysis done by [52] found out that episiotomy is associated with increased incidence and severity of postpartum perineal pain.

2. Conclusion

An episiotomy is, therefore, a traumatic procedure that should be practiced restrictively. World Health Organization (WHO) Guideline Developing Groups and FIGO emphasized the need for health systems to adopt a policy of restrictive rate of not more than 10%, and mediolateral episiotomy type is the one recommended, and this should be performed under adequate analgesia, whether anesthesia is already in place for labor, such as epidural, or by administering a local infiltration.

Conflict of interest

The authors declare no conflict of interest.

Author details

Francis Pebolo Pebalo* and Jackline Ayikoru
Faculty of Medicine, Department of Reproductive Health, Gulu University, Gulu, Uganda

*Address all correspondence to: pebalopebolo@gmail.com

References

[1] Usha DSSADV. A Clinical study of Agaruvadi Yoni Dhupana on episiotomy wound. European Journal of Biomedical and Pharmaceutical sciences. 2016;**3**(3):322-327

[2] Borruto FCC. Episiotomy: A too often unnecessary and harmful practice. MOJ Womens Health. 2016;**2**(1):00020

[3] Thacker SB, Banta HD. Benefits and risks of episiotomy: An interpretative review of the English language literature, 1860-1980. Obstetrical & Gynecological Survey. 1983;**38**(6):322-338

[4] Myers-Helfgott MG, Helfgott AW. Routine use of episiotomy in modern obstetrics. Should it be performed? Obstetrics and Gynecology Clinics of North America. 1999;**26**:305-325

[5] Gabbe SG. The prophylactic forceps operation 1920. American Journal of Obstetrics and Gynecology. 2002;**187**(255):254

[6] Amorim MM, Franca-Neto AH, Leal NV, Melo FO, Maia SB, Alves JN. Is it possible to never perform episiotomy during vaginal delivery? Obstetrics & Gynecology. 2014;**123**:38

[7] D'Gregorio P. Obstetric violence: A new legal term introduced in Venezuela. International Journal of Gynaecology and Obstetrics. 2010;**111**:201-202

[8] Nygaard CC et al. Appraisal of clinical practice guidelines on the management of obstetric perineal lacerations and care using the AGREE II instrument. European Journal of Obstetrics, Gynecology, and Reproductive Biology. 2020;**247**:66-72

[9] Zaami S et al. Does episiotomy always equate violence in obstetrics? Routine and selective episiotomy in obstetric practice and legal questions. European Review for Medical and Pharmacological Sciences. 2019;**23**(5):1847-1854

[10] Fodstad K, Staff AC, Laine K. Effect of different episiotomy techniques on perineal pain and sexual activity 3 months after delivery. International Urogynecology Journal. 2014;**25**(12):1629-1637

[11] Kilpatrick S. Normal labor and Delivery in Obstetrics, Normal and Problem Pregnancies. 5th ed. P.C.L. Amsterdam, Netherlands: Elsevier; 2007

[12] Kettle CHR, Ismail KM. Continuous versus interrupted sutures for repair of episiotomy or second degree tears. Cochrane Database of Systematic Reviews. 2012;**4**:11

[13] Sagi-Dain L. Morbidity associated with episiotomy in vacuum delivery: A systematic review and meta-analysis. An International Journal of Obstetrics & Gynaecology. 2015;**122**:1073-1081

[14] WHO. WHO Recommendations for Prevention and Treatment of Maternal Peripartum Infections. Geneva, Switzerland, WHO; 2015

[15] Graham Ian D et al. Episiotomy rates around the world: An update. Birth. 2005;**32**(3):219-223

[16] Wright A et al. FIGO good clinical practice paper: Management of the second stage of labor. International Journal of Gynaecology and Obstetrics. 2021;**152**(2):172-181

[17] Tomasso G, Althabe F, Cafferata ML, Aleman A, Sosa C. The need to avoid the routine use of episiotomy. Current

Women's Health Reviews. 2006;**2**:99-102. DOI: 10.2174/157340406776931034

[18] Frankman EA, Bunker CH, et al. Episiotomy in the United States; has anything changed? American Journal of Obstetrics and Gynecology. 2009; **200**:573.e1-573.e7

[19] Eltorkey MM, Eltorkey MM, Al Nuaim MA, Kurdi AM, Sabagh TO, Clarke F. Episiotomy, elective or selective: A report of a random allocation trial. Journal of Obstetrics and Gynaecology. 1994;**14**:317-320

[20] Clesse C et al. Episiotomy practices in France: Epidemiology and risk factors in non-operative vaginal deliveries. Scientific Reports. 2020;**10**(1):20208

[21] Goueslard K et al. How did episiotomy rates change from 2007 to 2014? Population-based study in France. BMC Pregnancy and Childbirth. 2018;**18**(1):208

[22] Goh R, Goh D, Ellepola H. Perineal tears—A review. The Australian Journal of General Practice. 2018;**47**(1-2):35-38

[23] Chigbu BOS, Alukaa Kamanu C, Adibe E. Factors influencing the use of episiotomy in Nigeria, should their use be restricted? Nigerian Postgraduate Medical Journal. 2008;**1**(9):13-16

[24] Barnabas TAI, Olusyo A, Amale DA. Relative frequency and predictors of episiotomy in Ogbomoso Nigeria. Internat Journal of Medical Update. 2012;**7**(2):41-44

[25] Carvalho CC, Moraes FO. Pernambuco. Prevalence and factors associated with practice of episiotomy at a maternity school in Recife. Med Bras. 2010;**56**(3):333-339

[26] Geranmayeh M et al. Reducing perineal trauma through perineal massage with vaseline in second stage of labor. Archives of Gynecology and Obstetrics. 2012;**285**(1):77-81

[27] Shahoei R et al. The effect of perineal massage during the second stage of birth on nulliparous women perineal: A randomization clinical trial. Electronic Physician. 2017;**9**(10):5588-5595

[28] Akhlaghi F et al. Effect of perineal massage on the rate of episiotomy. Journal of Family & Reproductive Health. 2019;**13**(3):160-166

[29] Labrecque M et al. Randomized controlled trial of prevention of perineal trauma by perineal massage during pregnancy. American Journal of Obstetrics & Gynecology. 1999;**180**(3):593-600

[30] West Z, Isaacs L. In:. West Z, Isaacs L. editiors. Chapter 10—Preparation for labour, in Acupuncture in Pregnancy and Childbirth. 2nd edition. Edinburgh: Churchill Livingstone; 2008. p. 155-168

[31] Kavvadias T, Hoesli I. The EpiNo® device: Efficacy, tolerability, and impact on pelvic floor—Implications for future research. Obstetrics and Gynecology International. 2016;**2016**:3818240-3818240

[32] Lincová M et al. Obstetric anal sphincter injuries - review of our date between 2015-2017. Ceská Gynekologie. 2019;**84**(1):18-22

[33] Fernando RJ, Adams EJ. RCOG Green Top Guidelines: Management of Third and Fourth Degree Perineal Tears Following Vaginal Delivery. Green Top Guidelines; 2007

[34] Keriakos R, Gopinath D. Obstetric anal sphincter injuries. Journal of Acute Disease. 2015;**4**(4):259-265

[35] Varma A, Gunn J, Gardiner A, Lindow SW, Duthie GS. Obstetric anal sphincter injury. Diseases of the Colon & Rectum. 1999;**42**(12):1537-1542

[36] Kapoor DS, Thakar R, Sultan AH. Obstetric anal sphincter injuries: Review of anatomical factors and modifiable second stage *interventions*. International Urogynecology Journal. 2015;**26**(12):1725-1734

[37] van Roon YKC, Rahman N, Vinayakarao L, Melson L, Kester N, Pathak S, et al. Comparison of obstetric anal sphincter injuries in nulliparous women before and after introduction of the EPISCISSORS-60® at two hospitals in the United Kingdom. International Journal of Women's Health. 2015;7:949-955

[38] Jansson MH et al. Risk factors for perineal and vaginal tears in primiparous women—The prospective POPRACT-cohort study. BMC Pregnancy and Childbirth. 2020;**20**(1):749

[39] Spinelli A et al. Diagnosis and treatment of obstetric anal sphincter injuries: New evidence and perspectives. Journal of Clinical Medicine. 2021;**10**(15):3261

[40] Fernando RSA, Kettle C, Thakar R. Methods of repair for obstetric anal sphincter injury. Cochrane Database of Systematic Reviews. 2013;**12**:CD002866

[41] Napoé GS, Foust-Wright CE, Pulliam SJ, Melamed A, Batalden RP, Berkowitz LR. Confidence in repair of obstetric anal sphincter injuries and objective assessment in obstetricians. Practice. 2015;**20**(20):24-24

[42] Zilberman A et al. Once episiotomy, always episiotomy? Archives of Gynecology and Obstetrics. 2018;**298**(1):121-124

[43] Viswanathan M, Hartmann K, Palmieri R, Lux L, Swinson T, Lohr KN, et al. The Use of Episiotomy in Obstetrical Care: A Systematic Review: Summary. Rockville, Maryland: AHRQ Evidence Report Summaries; 2005

[44] Alum AC et al. Factors associated with early resumption of sexual intercourse among postnatal women in Uganda. Reproductive Health. 2015;**12**(1):107

[45] Woolley RJ. Benefits and risks of episiotomy: A review of the English-language literature since 1980, Part I. Obstetrical & Gynecological Survey. 1995;**50**(11):806-820

[46] El-Nagger MHA. Effect of self perineal care instructions on episiotomy pain and wound healing of postpartum women. Journal of American Science. 2012;**8**(6):640-650

[47] Davidson. REEDA: Evaluating postpartum healing. Journal of Nurse-Midwifery. 1974;**19**:6-9

[48] Pebolo PF, Judith A, Dan KK. Episiotomy related morbidities measured using redness, edema, ecchymosis, discharge and apposition scale and numerical pain scale among primiparous women in Mulago National Referral Hospital, Kampala, Uganda. The Pan African Medical Journal. 2020;**36**:347

[49] Odar E, Wandabwa J, Kiondo P. Sexual practices of women within six months of childbirth in Mulago hospital, Uganda. African Health Sciences. 2003;**3**(3):117-123

[50] Woolley RJ. Benefits and risks of episiotomy: A review of the English-language literature since 1980, Part II. Obstetrical & Gynecological Survey. 1995;**50**:820-835

[51] Amorim M et al. Selective episiotomy vs. implementation of a non-episiotomy protocol: A randomized clinical trial. Reproductive Health. 2017;**14**(1):55

[52] Gün İ, Doğan B, Özdamar Ö. Long- and short-term complications of episiotomy. Turkish Journal of Obstetrics and Gynecology. 2016;**13**(3):144-148

Chapter 5

Recent Advances in the Use of Uterotonics for the Prevention of Postpartum Hemorrhage

Rajasri G. Yaliwal

Abstract

Primary postpartum hemorrhage (PPH) is one of the leading causes of maternal morbidity and mortality worldwide. The most common cause of primary PPH is uterine atony. Various uterotonics have been used over the years for the prevention of PPH. Oxytocin, Ergometrine, Misoprostol, and Carboprost have been extensively studied. Recently, Carbetocin, an analog of Oxytocin has been added to the armamentarium of postpartum hemorrhage. However, the optimal route and dose of these drugs are still being studied. Oxytocin induces superior myometrial contractions when compared with Ergometrine, Carboprost and Misoprostol. The effect of Oxytocin is reduced in myometrium of women with Oxytocin-augmented labor; however, it is still superior to the other uterotonics. Although the value of universal use of uterotonics to reduce postpartum hemorrhage after vaginal birth has been well established, their value in cesarean section has received little attention. It has been assumed that the benefits of oxytocics observed at vaginal birth also apply to cesarean section. The route of Oxytocin has been studied by various researchers. Intravenous (IV) infusion of Oxytocin has been preferred during cesarean section as an IV line would have been already secured and it has faster plasma peak concentration as in comparison to the Intramuscular (IM) route. Though IV bolus Oxytocin has been associated with a faster peak plasma concentration of Oxytocin, faster uterine contraction; it also has been associated with sudden hypotension. Carbetocin is also another promising drug. It has been prioritized due to its heat stable and long-acting properties. It also reduces the need for infusions. It is still an expensive drug in many countries. Carbetocin is administered as 100 mcg IM/IV/IV infusion. The dose in elective cesarean may be less as shown in some studies. Misoprostol by oral route has been recommended by WHO at 400–600 mcg in places where Oxytocin cannot be administered. Syntometrine has lesser blood loss compared to Oxytocin alone.

Keywords: blood loss, oxytocics, oxytocin, carbetocin, ergometrine, carboprost, sulprostone, tranexamic acid, ethamsylate, cesarean, vaginal delivery

1. Introduction

Post-partum hemorrhage (PPH) is a devastating condition causing severe maternal morbidity and mortality. Uterine atonicity is the commonest cause of PPH and in turn, PPH is the commonest cause of maternal death across the continents. Though there are many predisposing factors for uterine atony, many a time it is unpredictable.

Postpartum hemorrhage is defined as blood loss of more than 500 ml after vaginal delivery and more than 1000 ml after cesarean delivery within 24 hours of childbirth.

Though the upper limits to define PPH have been established, the average blood loss during vaginal and cesarean delivery is much less. In a study conducted in France, which included 7908 participants, it was found that the mean blood loss after vaginal delivery was 180.1 mL (± 224.7 mL) and Cesarean delivery was 557.9 mL (± 496.2 mL) [1]. In another study conducted in rural India, the mean blood loss following delivery was 304 ml (range 50–975 ml). This was measured by Brass V drape [2]. Active management of third stage of labor (AMTSL) with the use of prophylactic uterotonics has reduced the incidence of PPH. However, based on evidence the World Health Organization (WHO) now considers controlled cord traction and uterine massage as optional. Delayed cord clamping is preferred. The only component of AMTSL which has been advocated is the use of uterotonic [3].

1.1 Oxytocin receptors

Endogenous Oxytocin is secreted by the paraventricular and supraoptic nuclei of the Hypothalamus. It stimulatesuterine contractions. Oxytocin receptors (OTR) are present not only in the uterus but also in other tissues namely limbic regions of the brain, spinal column, heart, intestines, immune tissue, uterus, and breast. The OTR belongs to a family of G Proteins coupled receptors [4].

The number of receptors over the uterus is low in the first trimester and increases gradually in the third trimester. They then reduce in number in the immediate postpartum period.

The lower segment also has a lower concentration of OTR in comparison to the funds of the uterus, while the cervix has the least concentration [5].

1.2 Cesarean versus vaginal delivery

The cesarean section brings about a varied situation in comparison to vaginal delivery. It could be done during active labor as in emergency cesarean section or when the woman is not in labor as in elective cesarean section. There is no consensus on the dose of Oxytocin in elective cesarean sections in comparison to cesareans done in active labor. The required dose of Oxytocin during elective cesarean section is less than the dose required during cesarean section done during active labor, however, there is no consensus about using a reduced dose. The guidelines for use of prophylactic uterotonics for vaginal delivery are being used for cesarean delivery. There are no specific guidelines for the use of uterotonics for cesarean delivery [6, 7]. Oxytocin may be required to be continued as an infusion for 2–4 hours after the commencement of administration for women undergoing cesarean section [8].

2. Uterotonics

Uterotonics have been used over the decades for both prophylaxis and treatment of PPH. The uterotonics are Oxytocin, Carbetocin, Ergometrine/Methyl ergometrine, Carboprost, Misoprostol, Dinoprostone, and Sulprostone. Combination of Oxytocin and methylergometrine are also used.

2.1 Oxytocin

The WHO recommends the use of Oxytocin as the first-choice prophylactic drug for the prevention of PPH. It can be used intramuscularly and when an intravenous line is in place, intravenously as an infusion. The recommended dose is 10 IU. It has a half-life of 1–6 minutes [9].

Various studies have used intravenous bolus of Oxytocin during cesarean and vaginal delivery.

Royal College of Obstetricians and Gynecologists (RCOG) guidelines recommend a bolus of 5 IU Oxytocin during cesarean delivery. Other studies have used doses as low as 1 IU and as high as 10 IU bolus during cesarean delivery. They have shown that Bolus Oxytocin did not have significant adverse effects as it was previously thought [10].

Intravenous bolus of 10 IU of Oxytocin has been used for the prevention of PPH during vaginal delivery. In a randomized control trial comparing intravenous bolus of 10 IU Oxytocin to intramuscular Oxytocin of 10 IU for prevention of PPH during vaginal delivery conducted in the Republic of Ireland, it was found that the incidence of PPH was lower in women administered intravenous bolus of Oxytocin in comparison to the intramuscular group (4.6 vs. 8.1%) [11]. In another large three-arm randomized control trial conducted in Egypt, comparing 10 IU of Oxytocin by intramuscular, intravenous bolus, and intravenous infusion, it was observed that the blood loss in the intravenous infusion group was 5.9% lesser than that occurring in the intramuscular group. The intravenous bolus group had 11.1% less blood loss in comparison to the intramuscular group. There were no significant differences in the adverse effects of Oxytocin among the three groups [12]. Intravenous bolus Oxytocin is shown to be a promising choice of uterotonic for the prevention of PPH without any significant adverse effects.

2.2 Carbetocin

Heat stable Carbetocin is a long-acting synthetic analog of Oxytocin. It has the benefit of being heat stable in comparison to the heat-sensitive Oxytocin. It does not require cold storage and has a good shelf life of 36 months at 30°C [13]. It is long acting having a half-life of 40 minutes. It is given in the dose of 100 mcg. Intramuscular, intravenous infusion, and intravenous bolus routes have been administered. Carbetocin, like Oxytocin, causes hypotension, tachycardia, and myocardial ischemia. It acts by 2 minutes of administration when given intravenously or intramuscularly [14–16]. The Champions trial conducted over 23 countries at 10 sites compared 100 mcg of Carbetocin to 10 IU of Oxytocin both given intramuscularly. It concluded that Carbetocin was noninferior to Oxytocin for the prevention of PPH and there was no significant difference between the adverse effects on both the groups [13].

It has now been recommended for prevention of PPH by the WHO [9]. It has not been recommended for therapeutic use in PPH. Carbetocin is for single use, it cannot be repeated. This is because it causes adverse effects with higher doses.

2.3 Misoprostol

This is a prostaglandin E1 analogue. It has the advantage of being in a tablet form and does not need refrigeration. It also has a long shelf life of 2–3 years [17]. It can be administered by oral, sublingually, buccal, vaginal, and rectally. Oral and sublingual route administration act faster than the vaginal and rectal routes. The overall serum concentration of buccal route is low. It has a half-life of 20–40 minutes [18]. A common practice is to moisten the Misoprostol prior to placing it vaginally. This has been found not to have any additional benefit in comparison to placing the tablet as it is [19].

Various doses and routes have been recommended for prophylaxis. Misoprostol 400 mcg and 600 mcg by oral route have been recommended by the WHO. According to a meta-analysis by the Cochrane database, the use of Misoprostol as a first-line agent may have increased blood loss in comparison to Oxytocin [20]. Adverse effects of shivering, diarrhea, and vomiting, though not life-threatening, can be worrisome for the patient [9].

2.4 Ergometrine and methyl ergometrine

Ergometrine and Methyl ergometrine i.e., the semi-synthetic form of ergometrine are long-acting uterotonic agents [21]. The onset of action is 2–3 minutes and the half-life is 30–120 minutes [9].

They act on the adrenergic and serotonin receptors on the uterus. It is given in the dose of 0.2 mg and can be administered by both IV and IM routes [22]. Ergot derivates are known to have severe cardiovascular adverse effects like hypertension, tachycardia, myocardial ischemia, and infarction. They can also cause cerebrovascular accidents and demise. For these reasons, it is not used as a first-line drug for prevention of PPH. It is not recommended in those women who suffer from hypertensive disorders of pregnancy or cardiac disease.

2.5 Carboprost tromethamine

Carboprost tromethamine is the synthetic 15-methyl analogue of prostaglandin $F_{2\alpha}$. It is listed as a therapeutic drug for postpartum hemorrhage by the WHO [9]. It acts by increasing the intracellular calcium of the myometrial cells, which in turn enhances the myosin light-chain kinase activity and uterine contractions. This action is mediated via the Prostaglandin F receptor which is a G protein-coupled receptor in the myometrium [23]. Carboprost is administered as 250 mcg intramuscular injection. It can be given as an intramyometrial injection as well. However, this is an off-label route. It cannot be given intravenously. It has a half-life of 8 minutes and its action peaks by 15–30 minutes. It is mainly used as a second line of treatment of postpartum hemorrhage. It is associated with gastrointestinal adverse effects, such as vomiting and diarrhea. It can also cause bronchospasm and is contraindicated in asthmatics [22]. Due to its adverse effects, it is not recommended by the WHO for prevention of postpartum hemorrhage [9].

2.6 Sulprostone

Sulprostone is a derivative of Prostaglandin E2 and acts on the PGEP3 receptor of the myometrium. It has been used for the treatment of PPH. It is used as an intravenous infusion. The dose is 100 mcg/hr. and can be given at 500 mcg/hr. dose. It is contraindicated in bronchial asthma.

According to the French College of Gynecologist and Obstetricians, Sulprostone is the second-line drug to be used in case there is a failure of Oxytocin in the management of postpartum hemorrhage [24]. This drug is used in European countries and is not available in US and Australia. It is not available in India either.

2.7 Combination of uterotonics

The combination of Methylergometrine 500 mcg and Oxytocin 5 IU, commonly known as Syntometrine, is used in some countries. It acts for 2.5 minutes and has a prolonged action of 3 hours. It is administered intramuscularly [9]. Though it has more adverse effects than Oxytocin alone like nausea, vomiting, and diarrhea, it is more effective in preventing PPH [25].

2.8 Misoprostol and oxytocin

This combination of oral misoprostol with intravenous/intramuscular Oxytocin aims to take the benefit of the fast-acting Oxytocin and the longer-acting misoprostol. Though the combination is promising, it is associated with more adverse effects of shivering, fever, nausea, vomiting, and diarrhea, in comparison to Oxytocin alone [9].

3. Hemostatic drugs: tranexamic acid and ethamsylate

Antifibrinolytic drugs can reduce blood loss during delivery. Tranexamic acid is an antifibrinolytic drug. It binds to plasminogenmolecule and bocks the lysin binding sites. It is administered intravenously as 1 gm after the administration of the prophylactic uterotonic.

Ethamsylate is another hemostatic drug that acts on the platelets and enhances their aggregation. It also improves capillary resistance. It is used as a 1 g intravenous dose. It can cause rash, nausea, vomiting, and hypotension [26, 27].

3.1 Estimation of blood loss after delivery

The diagnosis of postpartum hemorrhage itself can be challenging. The various methods commonly used to estimate the blood loss are the visual estimation of the blood loss, use of a funnel-shaped drape with an attached plastic sheet placed underneath the buttocks of the woman, otherwise known as the Excellent BRASS-V drape in which the blood collects, spectrophotometry and estimation of Hemoglobin concentration in the venous blood [28]. Other indirect methods include weighing soaked gauze pieces, mops and drapes, and adding blood collected in bowls and suction jars. The weight of the unsoaked mops and gauze pieces and drapes should be known.
1 g increase in the weight of the soaked material = 1 ml of blood [29].

An easier, quick, and efficient method to estimate the blood loss and to help in predicting the prognosis would be to use the Shock Index(SI). This is a simple bedside calculation using the ratio of heart rate (HR) and systolic blood pressure (SBP) [30].

$$SI = HR / SBP. \quad (1)$$

The normal SI range is 0.7–0.9 in pregnancy which is slightly higher than the non-pregnant SI which ranges from 0.5 to 0.7 [31]. If the SI is more than 1, it indicates cardiac decompensation and demands immediate treatment [32]. SI has been used to triage patients for referral, especially in low-resource settings. A value of $\geq$0.9 would suggest referring the patient to a tertiary care center, ≥1.4 immediate intervention, and ≥ 1.7 adverse prognosis [33].

3.2 Choosing the right uterotonic

With multiple uterotonics to choose from, selecting the appropriate one demands knowledge of the contraindications and adverse effects of the specific drug.

According to the WHO guidelines for the management of PPH, uterotonics are to be used in the following order.

First line of treatment: Oxytocin is the first-line drug to be used. It is to be used in dose of 20 IU in 1 liter of fluid at 40 drops per minute. It should not exceed 3 liters.

Second line of treatment: If not responding to this treatment, or if oxytocin is not available then, ergometrine or fixed-dose ergometrine and oxytocin can be used as second-line treatment of PPH. Methyl ergometrine can be given 0.2 mg IM or IV, it can be repeated after 4 hours and a maximum of 5 doses can be given.

Third line of treatment: Prostaglandins can be used as third-line drug if the patient does not respond to the previous treatments. Carboprostcan is given as 0.25 mg IM and can be repeated every 15 minutes for a maximum of 8 doses [9].

4. Conclusion

Oxytocin is the first-choice drug for the prevention of postpartum hemorrhage.

Carbetocin is a heat stable, longer-acting uterotonic which can be used in places where the cold chain and cold storage cannot be assured. However, it is expensive in comparison to Oxytocin.

Misoprostol is a heat-stable tablet that can be used if Oxytocin is unavailable. However, it is likely to be inferior to Oxytocin in the prevention of PPH.

Carboprost, though effective in controlling blood loss after the delivery, is used for therapeutic purposes than prophylaxis due to its adverse effects. It also requires refrigeration.

Ergot derivatives are second-like choices as they have cardiovascular adverse effects. It also requires refrigeration.

Sulprostone though considered as second-line drug for PPH in France and other European counties, is not available in many places.

Combination of drugs Misoprostol and Oxytocin or Syntometrine, while potentially reducing blood loss, seem to have more adverse effects; thus, administering Oxytocin alone is more advantageous.

Acknowledgements

I would like to thank Bijapur Lingayat District Education Deemed to be University (BLDE DU), Vijayapura, Karnataka, India for their continuous encouragement and support.

Conflict of interest

The authors declare no conflict of interest.

Financial disclosure

None.

Author details

Rajasri G. Yaliwal
Department of Obstetrics and Gynecology, BLDE (DU) Shri BM Patil Medical College, Hospital and Research Center, Vijayapura, Karnataka, India

*Address all correspondence to: ryaliwal@bldedu.ac.in

References

[1] Misme H, Dupont C, Cortet M, Rudigoz RC, Huissoud C. Analyse descriptive du volume des pertes sanguines au cours de l'accouchement par voie basse et par césarienne [Distribution of blood loss during vaginal delivery and cesarean section]. Journal de Gynecologie, Obstetrique et Biologie de la Reproduction. 2016;**45**(1):71-79. DOI: 10.1016/j.jgyn.2015.01.004

[2] Patel A, Goudar SS, Geller SE, et al. Drape estimation vs. visual assessment for estimating postpartum hemorrhage. International Journal of Gynaecology and Obstetrics. 2006;**93**(3):220-224. DOI: 10.1016/j.ijgo.2006.02.014. [published correction appears in Int J Gynaecol Obstet. 2006 Dec;95(3):312]

[3] WHO. Active management of the third stage of labour. June 2014

[4] Bell AF, Erickson EN, Carter CS. Beyond labor: The role of natural and synthetic oxytocin in the transition to motherhood. Journal of Midwifery & Women's Health. 2014;**59**(1):35-108. DOI: 10.1111/jmwh.12101

[5] Fuchs AR, Fuchs F, Husslein P, Soloff MS. Oxytocin receptors in the human uterus during pregnancy and parturition. American Journal of Obstetrics and Gynecology. 1984;**150**(6):734-741. DOI: 10.1016/0002-9378(84)90677-x

[6] Elbourne DR, Prendiville WJ, Carroli G, Wood J, McDonald S. Prophylactic use of Oxytocin in the third stage of labor. Cochrane Database System Review. 2001;**4**:CD001808

[7] Lokugamage AU, Paine M, Bassaw Balroop K, Sullivan KR, Refaey HE, Rodeck CH. Active management of the third stage at caesarean section: A randomised controlled trial of misoprostol versus syntocinon. The Australian & New Zealand Journal of Obstetrics & Gynaecology. 2001;**41**: 411-414. DOI: 10.1111/j.1479-828X.2001.tb01319.x

[8] Heesen M, Carvalho B, Carvalho JCA, et al. International consensus statement on the use of uterotonic agents during caesarean section. Anaesthesia. 2019;**74**(10):1305-1319. DOI: 10.1111/anae.14757

[9] WHO. WHO Recommendations: Uterotonics for the Prevention of Postpartum Haemorrhage. Geneva: World Health Organization; 2018

[10] Munn MB, Owen J, Vincent R, Wakefield M, Chestnut DH, Hauth JC. Comparison of two Oxytocin regimens to prevent uterine atony at cesarean delivery: A randomized controlled trial. Obstetrics and Gynecology. 2001;**98**:386-390

[11] Adnan N, Conlan-Trant R, McCormick C, Boland F, Murphy DJ. Intramuscular versus intravenous Oxytocin to prevent postpartum haemorrhage at vaginal delivery: Randomised controlled trial. BMJ. 2018;**362**:k3546. DOI: 10.1136/bmj.k3546

[12] Charles D, Anger H, Dabash R, et al. Intramuscular injection, intravenous infusion, and intravenous bolus of Oxytocin in the third stage of labor for prevention of postpartum hemorrhage: A three-arm randomized control trial. BMC Pregnancy Childbirth. 2019;**19**(1):38. DOI: 10.1186/s12884-019-2181-2

[13] Widmer M, Piaggio G, Nguyen TMH, et al. Heat-stable Carbetocin versus

oxytocin to prevent hemorrhage after vaginal birth. The New England Journal of Medicine. 2018;**379**(8):743-752. DOI: 10.1056/NEJMoa1805489

[14] Larciprete G, Montagnoli C, Frigo M, et al. Carbetocin versus oxytocin in caesarean section with high risk of post-partum haemorrhage. Journal of Perinatal Medicine. 2013;**7**(1):12-18

[15] WHO. World Health Organization Model List of Essential Medicines – 22nd List, 2021. Geneva: World Health Organization; 2021 (WHO/MHP/HPS/EML/2021.02). Licence: CC BY-NC-SA 3.0 IGO

[16] Cordovani D, Balki M, Farine D, Seaward G, Carvalho JC. Carbetocin at elective cesarean delivery: A randomized controlled trial to determine the effective dose. Canadian Journal of Anaesthesia. 2012;**59**(8):751-757. DOI: 10.1007/s12630-012-9728-2

[17] Hagen N, Khuluza F, Heide L. Quality, availability and storage conditions of oxytocin and misoprostol in Malawi. BMC Pregnancy Childbirth. 2020;**20**:184. DOI: 10.1186/s12884-020-2810-9

[18] Allen R, O'Brien BM. Uses of misoprostol in obstetrics and gynecology. Reviews in Obstetrics and Gynecology. 2009;**2**(3):159-168

[19] Tang OS, Schweer H, Seyberth HW, Lee SW, Ho PC. Pharmacokinetics of different routes of administration of misoprostol. Human Reproduction. 2002;**17**(2):332-336

[20] Parry Smith WR, Papadopoulou A, Thomas E, et al. Uterotonic agents for first-line treatment of postpartum haemorrhage: A network meta-analysis. Cochrane Database System Review. 2020;**11**(11):CD012754. DOI: 10.1002/14651858.CD012754.pub2

[21] Balki M, Wong CA. Refractory uterine atony: Still a problem after all these years. International Journal of Obstetric Anesthesia. 2021;**48**:103207. DOI: 10.1016/j.ijoa.2021.103207

[22] Fanning RA, Sheehan F, Leyden C, Duffy N, Iglesias-Martinez LF, Carey MF, Campion DP, O'Connor JJ. A role for adrenergic receptors in the uterotonic effects of ergometrine in isolated human term nonlaboring myometrium. Anesthesia & Analgesia. 1 May 2017;**124**(5):1581-1588

[23] PubChem [Internet]. Bethesda (MD): National Library of Medicine (US), National Center for Biotechnology Information; 2004-. PubChem Compound Summary for CID 5281074, Carboprost tromethamine; [cited 2022 Mar. 2]. Available from: https://pubchem.ncbi.nlm.nih.gov/compound/Carboprost-tromethamine

[24] Sentilhes L, Vayssière C, Deneux-Tharaux C, et al. Postpartum hemorrhage: Guidelines for clinical practice from the French College of Gynaecologists and Obstetricians (CNGOF): In collaboration with the French Society of Anesthesiology and Intensive Care (SFAR). European Journal of Obstetrics, Gynecology, and Reproductive Biology. 2016;**198**:12-21. DOI: 10.1016/j.ejogrb.2015.12.012

[25] Gallos ID, Williams HM, Price MJ, et al. Uterotonic agents for preventing postpartum haemorrhage: A network meta-analysis. Cochrane Database of Systematic Reviews. 2018;**4**(4):CD011689. Published 2018 Apr 25. DOI: 10.1002/14651858.CD011689.pub2

[26] Sentilhes L, Daniel V, Deneux-Tharaux C, et al. TRAAP2—TRAnexamic acid for preventing postpartum hemorrhage after cesarean delivery: A multicenter randomized, doubleblind, placebo- controlled trial – A study

protocol. BMC Pregnancy and Childbirth. 2020;**20**:63. DOI: 10.1186/s12884-019-2718-4

[27] Alanwar A, Gamal M. Tranexamic acid and Ethamsylate for reducing blood loss in patient undergoing lower segment cesarean section at high risk for post-partum hemorrhage: A pilot study. Open Journal of Obstetrics and Gynecology. 2020;**10**:1340-1350. DOI: 10.4236/ojog.2020.1090123

[28] Diaz V, Abalos E, Carroli G. Methods for blood loss estimation after vaginal birth. Cochrane Database System Review. 2018;**9**(9):CD010980. DOI: 10.1002/14651858.CD010980.pub2

[29] Ambardekar S, Shochet T, Bracken H, et al. Calibrated delivery drape versus indirect gravimetric technique for the measurement of blood loss after delivery: A randomized trial. BMC Pregnancy Childbirth. 2014;**14**:276. DOI: 10.1186/1471-2393-14-276

[30] Chaudhary M, Maitra N, Sheth T, Vaishnav P. Shock index in the prediction of adverse maternal outcome. Journal of Obstetrics and Gynaecology of India. 2020;**70**(5):355-359. DOI: 10.1007/s13224-020-01355-z

[31] Le BasChandraharan AE, Adie A, et al. Use of the "obstetrics shock index" as an adjunct in identifying significant blood loss in patients with massive post-partum hemorrhage. International Journal of Gynecology & Obstetrics. 2014;**124**:253-255. DOI: 10.1016/j.ijgo.2013.08.020

[32] Pacagnella RC, Borovac-Pinheiro A. Assessing and managing hypovolemic shock in puerperal women. Best Practice & Research. Clinical Obstetrics & Gynaecology. 2019;**61**:89-105. DOI: 10.1016/j.bpobgyn.2019.05.012

[33] El Ayadi AM, Nathan HL, Seed PT, et al. Vital sign prediction of adverse maternal outcomes in women with hypovolemic shock: The role of shock index. PLoS One. 2016;**11**(2):e0148729. DOI: 10.1371/journal.pone.0148729

Section 4

The New Born

Chapter 6

New Technologies to Dating Pregnancy at Birth

Zilma Silveira Nogueira Reis, Gabriela Silveira Neves and Roberta Maia de Castro Romanelli

Abstract

The chapter provides a vision of new methods of pregnancy dating at birth to overcome the high costs of existing approaches or lack of access to the existing technologies. The authors have presented a literature review on recent scientific reports exploring novel technologies, such as those based on the newborn's skin maturity assessment as machine learning models based on clinical data. The effortlessness of new approaches based on simplified clinical systems contrasting with molecular genetics and newborns screening analytes is discussed, even in scientific validation. Without the intention of an exhaustive or systematic review, we searched databases for reports concerning postnatal gestational age, prediction or estimate, novel approach, low and medium-income countries since 2015. Therefore, the authors did not compromise to offer a comprehensive picture of all postnatal gestational age methods. On the other hand, prematurity identification at birth remains a challenge in many birth settings, mainly in a scenario with scarce resources. Although postnatal pregnancy dating methods have strengths and disadvantages, this information is critical to recognize the risk of the newborn during the first hours of life, justifying technological investments.

Keywords: gestational age, infant, premature, skin physiological phenomena, artificial intelligence, equipment, and supplies

1. Introduction

The estimate of antenatal age faces the lacking of certainty of the day in the female cycle on which conception occurred and the dependence of early prenatal care access with crown-rump-length ultrasound measure [1]. While maternal-child worldwide policies do not provide a broad spectrum of technological options to obtain a reliable gestational age, the last menstrual period (LMP) remains the most extensive reference for pregnancy dating in many low and medium-income countries [2, 3]. However, a reliable last menstrual period (LMP) depends on sure of dates, regular cycles, absence of bleeding, or use of hormonal contraceptives in the last months before the date. In such a scenario, uncertainties related to memory bias, irregular menstrual cycles, breastfeeding, or failure of contraceptives have deprived many pregnant women and their babies of trustable gestational age [4]. The consequences are not restricted to antenatal care since prematurity identification at birth remains a challenge for neonatal care. Most of the preterm birth occurs in settings with limited resources to achieve a trustworthy chronology of gestation and, at the same time, neonatal due care. Preterm births and their complications are the leading cause of death of children under 5 years [5]. Most preterm births occur in the late preterm period, making decision-making difficult about what interventions and levels of assistance are needed [6]. Thus, gestational age is critical information to make timely decisions and provide appropriate neonatal support.

1.1 Disclosure agreement

The chapter provides a vision of new methods of pregnancy dating at birth to overcome the high costs of existing approaches or lack of access to the existing technologies, presenting recent scientific reports without an exhaustive or systematic review of the literature. We searched databases for reports concerning postnatal gestational age, prediction or estimate, novel approach, low and medium-income countries since 2015. Therefore, the authors did not compromise to offer a comprehensive picture of all postnatal gestational age methods. The authors have been working on solutions for gestational age prediction for scenarios with low resources and a scarcity of health facilities.

2. Technologies based on the newborn skin maturity

The skin barrier, formed during gestation, is essential for neonatal survival. It is not by coincidence that this essential protection exists since the limit of the viability of preterm infants means around 24 weeks [7]. However, the competence of the skin barrier against the loss of body heat and water ad infections depends on a process of maturity along the time. The analysis of the newborn's skin has shown a potential relation of the structure of this tissue with the chronology of gestation, reflecting the temporal process of skin maturation [8]. Part of the due care delivered to preterm newborns is a skin immaturity compensation as an incubator or a radiant warmer and environment humidity. It is not news that there are critical clinical connections between the competence of the skin barrier with the neonatal survival [9].

Markers of pregnancy dating from the newborn's skin are available by invasive and noninvasive technicians.

2.1 Invasive assessment: Histology

Microscopic images analysis is the basis of invasive approaches. The measurement of skin thickness is an important parameter that indirectly reflects the state of neonatal maturity and how prepared the newborn will be in the period of adaptation to the external environment [10]. Structural patterns that are strongly related to fetal age are easy to recognize as potential markers of skin maturation [10]. Structural patterns are strongly related to fetal age, are easy to recognize as potential markers of skin maturation [10]. **Figure 1** shows the skin of stillbirths from biopsies over the plantar surface of the sole at different gestational ages. The epidermis is the outermost layer, organized by stratified pavement epithelial tissue sublayers, which is keratinized in its external bound. Fetal epidermal thickness presents a clinical significance for the diagnosis of fetal prematurity [11, 12]. However, using measures with imaging software support, the

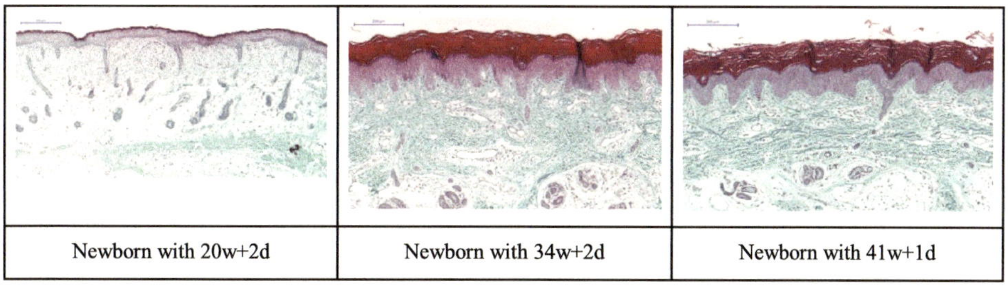

Figure 1.
Histological images of the skin over the sole of the foot. Note: Gomori trichrome staining, scale: 200 μm. Source: The authors.

composite formed by the thickness of the epidermis, dermis, and the area of sebaceous glands achieved an excellent correlation with gestational age ($r = 0.99$, $p < 0.001$) in dead concepts ranging from 20.3 to 41.6 weeks of gestation [11]. Meantime, the histological study of this tissue met limitations due to its invasive acquisition of materials from a human being for ethical issues [13]. Despite this, invasive postmortem studies can provide a basis for noninvasive approaches for alive newborns, at the same time provide information to support necropsies.

2.2 Noninvasive assessment of skin

Noninvasive assessment of skin maturity to predict gestational age is possible just as an overview impression or analyzing medical images. Moreover, a new technology reported gestational age correlation with optical properties of the newborn skin at birth [14]. An ongoing multicentric study has been conducted to validate this technology based on this proof of concept [15].

The skin characteristics have been used in several clinical scores for decades. Visible modifications during clinical ectoscopy of newborns have demonstrated that the skin of extremely premature has little or no visible pigmentation, being markedly erythematous, putting these and other characteristics of the skin as potential markers of the chronology of pregnancy, as provided by maturity scores [16, 17]. External characteristics of the newborn involving edema and skin opacity, lanugo, ear form, and firmness are antecedents in assessing gestational age at birth [18]. Besides, the composite anthropometric measurements, external characteristics, neurological tests, postnatal examination of epiphyseal center, and ulnar nerve motor conduction velocity are described, with 95% of the infants correctly estimated within ±3 weeks [19].

The melanin index is an optical skin parameter related to the melanin content in the tissue, accessible with bio-optical models [20], even in newborns [21]. The quantification of changes in skin reflection according to pigment distribution and concentration has been associated with gestational age, by using the melanin index [22] and the skin reflection by spectrophotometry [23]. Noninvasive approaches grounded on optics have the potential for characterization of the skin maturity, in addition to or in replacement of biopsy analysis. The advantages over histological techniques are keeping the original tissue morphology and providing *in vivo* tissue analysis, in real time.

An innovative multiband photometer was developed to assess gestational age at birth analyzing the skin transparency (**Figure 2**). This reflective test automatically processes the light, scattered by the skin against the device, when a small optoelectronic light emitter/receiver sensor touches the newborn's skin. A feasibility

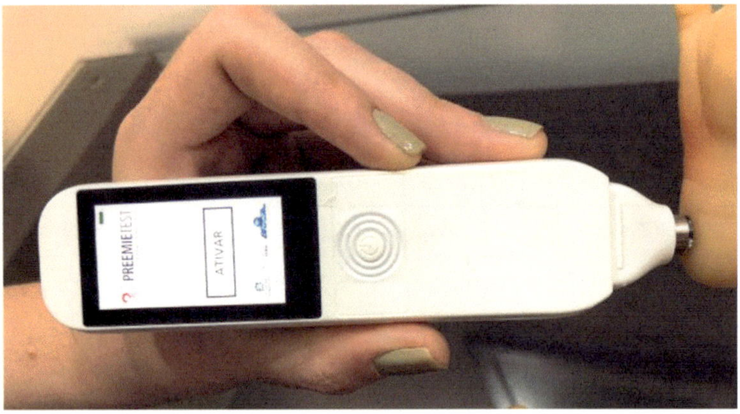

Figure 2.
The application of the multiband photometer for predict gestational age prediction in simulated newborn-doll application. Source: The authors.

study provided a mathematical model to predict gestational age based on the skin reflectance adjusted to clinical variables (R2 = 0.828, p < 0.001) [14]. A multicenter clinical trial evaluated the accuracy of this technology to detect preterm newborns, adding machine learning models to adjust birth weight and antenatal corticosteroid therapy for fetal maturation. For prematurity discrimination, the area under the receiver operating characteristic curve (AUROC) was 0.986 (95% CI: 0.977 to 0.994). Considering 7 days of error range, this device correctly detected 98.7% of gestational ages, preprint report of the author [10.21203/rs.3.rs-1,216,628/v2]. A new ongoing study to evaluate the device's ability to detect prematurity or small for gestational age, or both conditions simultaneously and predict short-term pulmonary complications in a cohort of low-birth-weight newborns has been conducted [24].

Another opportunity is assessing the skin of a newborn with dermatologic ultrasound equipment. The morphology of the skin can be observed *in vivo* with high-frequency ultrasonography. The microstructure of human skin is visualized in three layers and the skin thickness has a high correlation with that verified in histology from skin biopsies in adults (r = 0.96, p < 0.0001) [25]. Regarding the newborn's skin, Petersen et al. associated prematurity with the dermal and subcutaneous fat thickness obtained by ultrasonography on the plantar surface with the skinfold measure to support the nutritional evaluation in the neonatal period, analyzing echograms [26]. Vitral et al. analyzed 436 images of the skin in 222 newborns and reported a relationship between gestational age at birth to neonatal skin layer thickness obtained by ultrasound. Epidermal skin thickness on the forearm correlated with the gestational length, in the natural logarithm function (r = 0.610, p < 0.001). This parameter was not influenced by the standard of fetal growth as intrauterine growth restriction [27]. **Figure 3** shows three high-frequency ultrasonography images of the skin over the forearm of newborns of different gestational ages. A detailed protocol of the skin assessment with high-frequency ultrasound is available at dx.doi.org/10.17504/protocols.io.nfgdbjw.

Dermatologic ultrasound devices with high-frequency probe are portable and more economically accessible than conventional ultrasound. However, they are specific to skin evaluation and demand training [28].

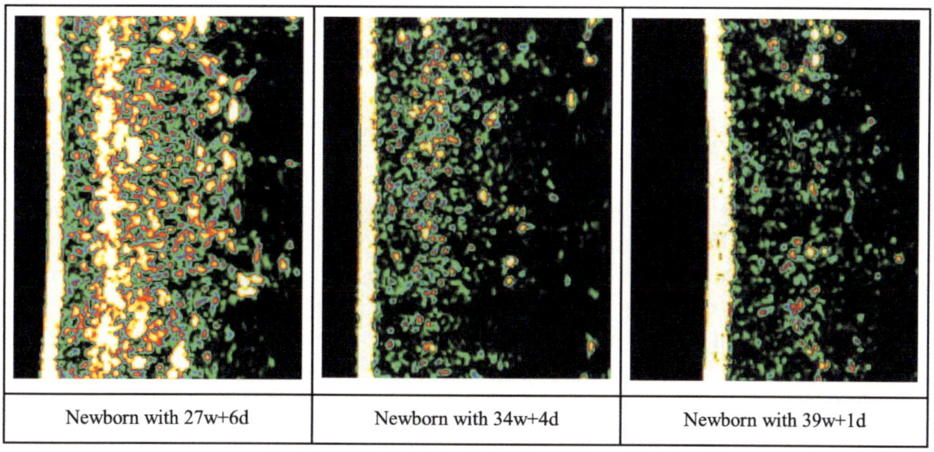

Figure 3.
High-frequency ultrasonography image of the skin over the forearm. Note: Epidermis corresponds to the white layer at the left side, resolution: 356- × 276-pixel. Source: The authors.

3. New approaches based on clinical characteristics

Novel methods based on clinical features for establishing an infant's gestational age have emerged that may be able to overcome some of the existing limitations.

3.1 The foot length

Measuring the postnatal foot length of the newborn is an alternative method for preterm newborn discrimination. Such an approach requires minimal training, is fast, and requires minimal handling. In addition, it causes wisp distress to premature infants or ill infants. Therefore, health professionals can use it with different levels of skills, making it applicable for a low-resource setting [29]. Using a plastic ruler, tape, or paper footprint, the accuracy of this measure for preterm newborns discrimination reached 76.9% sensitivity and 53.9% specificity [30]. The high inter-and intra-observer agreement is an advantage of this approach [31].

Furthermore, to underground this method, the foot length is an alternative for gestational age estimation during intrauterine life. It matters when other existent markers are unreliable, such as when the fetal is hydrocephalus, anencephaly, or limb dysplasia [31]. However, the strong correlation of fetal foot length with the chronology of gestational age, correlation coefficient $r = 0.960$, ($p < 0.001$), became from narrow results by small samples [32]. Limitations for this method are the influence of fetal growth, as foot measurements incorporate bone and soft tissue. Soft tissue stores of subcutaneous fat are decreased in small for gestational age infants and may be increased in large for gestational age infants, interfering with the accuracy of the test [31].

A recent study compared clinical examinations for gestational dating with a mask to the ultrasound-based gestational age at birth. Different approaches for pregnancy dating at birth are LMP, New Ballard (NBS), foot length, anterior lens assessments and anthropometric measures (including BW and birth length and mid-upper arm, abdominal and head circumferences measures at the time of assessment), and an

End-of-Bed gestational age assessment based on a brief nonstructured examination. Unfortunately, none of the methods studied could confidently predict the gestational age of individual babies within 1 week [33].

3.2 Simplified clinical score methods

End-of-Bed gestational age assessment itself concerns a simplified clinical score for newborn maturity. The development and tests were conducted in South Africa. Such non-structure evaluation presented lower bias in inter-observer agreement. However, it presented 2 weeks difference compared to reference early ultrasound [33].

Another approach based on clinical assessment is score methods, such as simplified gestational age score (SGAS). It was developed by using the most predictive items from the 12-item from NBS, 21-item Dubowitz score (DWS), and 11-item Meharban Singh (MS) and validated against the best obstetrics estimate in low-birth-weight newborns in India. The NBS, DWS, and MS were reduced to four, five, and six items, respectively, and all of them reduced total scores were not significantly different from the total score's estimate of gestational ($p > 0.05$). Such promising results and ease-to-use approach conducted to an adaptation to a mobile application, the T-SGAS, include a simple score associated with simple technology, using an app with combinations of references standards [34].

A cross-sectional validation study evaluated the accuracy of the mobile version of T-SGAS to ascertain postnatal gestational age within 24 hours of birth. A total of 8591 live singleton births whose gestational age by LMP and ultrasound was within 1 week of each other were enrolled. T-SGAS consisted of photographs that were the best fit for each score of the following four items: newborn's posture (score 0 to +4), skin (score − 1 to +5), breast (score − 1 to +4), and genitals (score − 1 to +4). The mobile app then auto-calculated the total score and classified the newborn's gestational age category. Such test showed strong inter-observer agreement (concordance correlation coefficient 0.77 (95% CI 0.76–0.78) and Fleiss' kappa was 0.76 (95% CI 0.76–0.78). ROC curves showed that the predictive accuracy of T-SGAS varied between 74% (LMP or USG) to 79% (LMP and USG). The simplicity of use by nurse-midwives has pointed it to be a helpful tool in resource-limited settings [34].

However, clinical maturity scores have presented lower values for small for gestational age infants and underestimated gestational age considering physical characteristics. Neurological evaluation is less affected by intrauterine growth and nutrition. Besides, they can be affected by infectious, metabolic, and other clinical conditions [35].

3.3 Cerebral maturity

Under visual or spectral analysis, the maturational electroencephalography (EEG) patterns of the newborn are associated with low development scores in small-for-gestational-age and low-birth-weight. This approach can reveal the delayed brain function development and not necessarily the gestational age [36].

4. Learning models for gestational age prediction at birth

Computer science has advanced detecting patterns by processing datasets through layered mathematical models, fostering skills and competencies of professionals to support the best healthcare decisions [37]. Machine learning models brought opportunities for data science to improve prediction models for pregnancy dating. Keeping the attention on postnatal gestational age estimative, a sort of reports associated variables to discriminate better preterm from term newborns.

A multicountry prospective study developed machine learning models to predict postnatal gestational age, gathering anthropometry, neuromuscular/physical signs, and feeding maturity variables. The most precise algorithm included infant sex, five anthropometric measurements, three physical and one neurological sign, and LMP, correctly classifying 91% of infants as preterm or term [38].

Another report on machine learning models relied on a set of options, including birth weight, LMP, and NBS, to estimate gestational age as a continuous outcome. The advantage is using variables accessible to health workers in resource-limited settings at the time of delivery, even without medical records. The correct classification of predictive models combining variables varied from 83.6% to 94.0% concerning NBS with LMP composite in parts or totally [39].

5. Newborn screening analytes to predict gestational age

Newborn screening programs are available worldwide with broad coverage, even using different protocols. Metabolic screening profiles have the potential for preventing severe health problems of newborns detecting different conditions at birth [40]. However, the newborn bloodspot screening commonly used to identify inborn errors of metabolism or other inherited disorders offers new opportunities to provide accurate estimates of gestational age [41].

There is considerable potential value in using metabolic markers to measure gestational age after birth. The newborn fetal/adult hemoglobin ratio provides gestational age estimative. Wilson et al., 2017 proposed a model for postnatal gestational age estimation utilizing newborn hemoglobin levels and metabolic analyte data derived from newborn blood spot samples. Models, including birth weight, hemoglobin, TSH, and 17-OHP levels, accurately estimated gestational age to ±2 weeks in 95·3% of the cohort and discriminated ≤34 versus >34 (c-statistic, 0·98) [42]. While models utilizing a full panel of newborn screening analytes accurately estimate gestational age, hemoglobin-based models are promising in discriminating ≥34 versus <34 weeks' gestational age, even where full mass spectrometry screening is not accessible [42].

Metabolites markers mirror metabolic processes during the first hour of life. There are many opportunities to assess newborn maturity using screening programs samples. The retrospective evaluation of the newborn screening dataset with infants from the different maternal origins in Ontario revealed distinct performance for gestational age prediction based on screening algorithm. It means that refining by development can predict gestational age better, and validation is necessary across the ethnicities [43]. Database from Iowa Newborn Screening Program considered 88 metabolites, and the models predicted gestational age within 1 week for 78% of neonates, with an area under the curve of 0.899 (95% confidence interval 0.895–0.903) in differentiating that born preterm (<37 weeks] from term (≥37 weeks) [44].

The advantages of this approach are drawn blood samples with minimum invasive for the newborn maturity evaluation, using cord blood and heel prick samples at birth. A predictive model including clinical data (infant sex, multiple births (yes/no), birth weight), screening analytes, and pairwise interactions had high accuracy in discriminating preterm from term newborns: AUROC 0.945 (95% CI 0.890, 0.999) for heel prick profiles and AUC 0.894 (95% CI 0.853, 0.935) for cord blood profiles [45].

Data from Newborn Screening Ontario (NSO) allowed for developing an algorithm capable of accurately estimating gestational age. Model performance was evaluated across multiple birth categories, such as ≥37, between 33 and 36, between 28 and 32, ≤27 weeks' gestation, ≤34, and < 37 weeks' gestational age. The algorithms estimated gestational age to be within 1.07 weeks of ultrasound-validated gestational age overall and correctly estimated gestational age to within 2 weeks for 94% of the infants. The validity in different ethnic populations showed outstanding performance although some variation in accuracy of gestational age estimation, 1.05 weeks among nonimmigrant mothers and 0.98 to 1.15 weeks among immigrant mothers. Moreover, aiming at low-income settings, the model was refined to facilitate its implementation where technological and resource requirements could be an issue. The ratio of fetal-to-adult Hb combined with clinical factors, such as sex and birth weight demonstrated better estimated gestational age than clinical covariates alone [46].

6. Molecular genetics in gestational age estimation

Gene expression has the potential to predict age-associated physiological changes. DNA methylation (DNAm) is associated with chronological age over long time scales and plays an essential role in development and growth. The mechanisms that drive changes in the aging methylome are not well understood; however, the quantitative measurements of methylome states may identify factors involved with slowed or accelerated aging rates [47].

DNAm of neonatal cord blood and blood spot samples has proven to accurately estimate gestational age at birth, from 24 to 44 weeks of gestation. The median absolute difference between DNAm gestational age and estimated clinical gestational age was 1.24 weeks, and the correlation coefficient was $r = 0.99$. It is a convenient molecular marker in that both exams are routinely performed to monitor neonatal health. Although DNAm demonstrated a remarkable correlation to estimated clinical gestational age, concerns whether gestational age acceleration is truly a measure of maturity versus a reflection of the relative accuracy of DNAm gestational age remains. Accurate classification systems that reflect both developmental time and maturity may improve the ability to predict neonatal risk [48].

Concerning studies of DNAm association to birth weight and chronological age, using cord blood, methylation at 224 CpG sites was found to be associated with gestational age and 23 CpG sites with birth weight [49]. There was a strong positive association between birth weight and development and a negative relationship between methylation and development in 12 of the 14 phenotypes. Of the 14 associations, eight involved methylations at cg15783941 (NFIX), and five were found in two CpG sites in the LTA gene [49].

7. Final considerations

The length of pregnancy has been estimated worldwide with the gestational age calculation at birth, using different available technologies. In childbirth settings, health professionals need gestational age assessment to make timely decisions to deliver newborn care and obtain vital statistics for public policies planning. Indeed, gestational age is a covariate in many studies and systems of the newborn's classification. All current methods have strengths and weaknesses, challenging recent technological advancements [49]. Prematurity identification remains a challenge in many birth settings, mainly in a scenario with scarce resources. There are promising novel approaches in different stages of development to provide a more easily obtainable and reliable gestational age. Developing new approaches under the vision of low-cost technologies are required to achieve birth settings in low and medium-income countries where pregnancy dating is more frequently unknown or absent.

Acknowledgements

This report is funded by Fundação Oswaldo Cruz – Rio de Janeiro, Brazil (Grant VPPIS-002-FEX-20.), Grand Challenges Canada' programs, Government of Canada –Toronto, Canada (Grant No. R-ST-POC-1807-13515). ZSNR is a researcher with scholarship from the Conselho Nacional de Desenvolvimento Científico e Tecnológico (CNPq – Brazil). The funders played no role in the study design, data collection, and analysis, decision to publish, or manuscript preparation.

Conflict of interest

Authors declare two patents deposit on behalf of the Universidade Federal de Minas Gerais and Fundação de Amparo a Pesquisa de Minas Gerais, Brazil, http://www.fapemig.br/en/, nonprofit institutions. The first author, ZSNR is one of the inventors for both BR1020170235688, and BR1020200215736.

Author details

Zilma Silveira Nogueira Reis[1,2,3]*, Gabriela Silveira Neves[3] and Roberta Maia de Castro Romanelli[1,3]

1 Faculty of Medicine, Center of Health Informatics, Universidade Federal de Minas Gerais, Belo Horizonte, Brazil

2 Faculty of Medicine, Department of Gynecology and Obstetrics, Universidade Federal de Minas Gerais, Belo Horizonte, Brazil

3 Faculty of Medicine, Postgraduate program in Child and Adolescent Health, Universidade Federal de Minas Gerais, Belo Horizonte, Brazil

*Address all correspondence to: zilma@ufmg.br

References

[1] Committee on Obstetric Practice tAIoUiM, and the Society for Maternal-Fetal Medicine. Committee opinion No 700: Methods for estimating the due date. Obstetrics and Gynecology. 2017;**129**(5):e150-e1e4. DOI: 10.1097/AOG.0000000000002046

[2] Lansky S, de Lima Friche AA, da Silva AAM, Campos D, de Azevedo Bittencourt SD, de Carvalho ML, et al. Pesquisa Nascer no Brasil: perfil da mortalidade neonatal e avaliação da assistência à gestante e ao recém-nascido Birth in Brazil survey: neonatal mortality profile, and maternal and child care. Cadernos de Saúde Pública. 2014;**30**:192-207. DOI: 10.1590/0102-311X00133213

[3] Scott K, Gupta S, Williams E, Arthur M, Somayajulu UV, Noguchi L. "I can guess the month ... but beyond that, I can't tell" an exploratory qualitative study of health care provider perspectives on gestational age estimation in Rajasthan, India. BMC Pregnancy and Childbirth. 2020;**20**(1):529. DOI: 10.1186/s12884-020-03201-6

[4] Karl S, Li Wai Suen CS, Unger HW, Ome-Kaius M, Mola G, White L, et al. Preterm or not--an evaluation of estimates of gestational age in a cohort of women from rural Papua New Guinea. PLoS One. 2015;**10**(5):e0124286. DOI: 10.1371/journal.pone.0124286

[5] Howson CP, Kinney MV, McDougall L, Lawn JE, Group BTSPBA. Born too soon: Preterm birth matters. Reproductive Health. 2013;**10**(Suppl. 1):S1. DOI: 10.1186/1742-4755-10-S1-S1

[6] Chawanpaiboon S, Vogel JP, Moller AB, Lumbiganon P, Petzold M, Hogan D, et al. Global, regional, and national estimates of levels of preterm birth in 2014: A systematic review and modelling analysis. The Lancet Global Health. 2019;**7**(1):e37-e46. DOI: 10.1016/S2214-109X(18)30451-0

[7] Hardman MJ, Moore L, Ferguson MW, Byrne C. Barrier formation in the human fetus is patterned. Journal of Investigative Dermatology. 1999;**113**(6):1106-1113

[8] Telofski LS, Morello AP, Mack Correa MC, Stamatas GN. The infant skin barrier: Can we preserve, protect, and enhance the barrier? Dermatology Research and Practice. 2012;**2012**:1-18. DOI: 10.1046/j.1523-1747.1999.00800.x

[9] Oranges T, Dini V, Romanelli M. Skin physiology of the neonate and infant: Clinical implications. Advances in Wound Care. 2015;**4**(10):587-595. DOI: 10.1089/wound.2015.0642

[10] Ersch J, Stallmach T. Assessing gestational age from histology of fetal skin: An autopsy study of 379 fetuses. Obstetrics & Gynecology. 1999;**94**(5, Part 1):753-757. DOI: 10.1016/s0029-7844(99)00379-8

[11] de Souza IMF, Vitral GLN, Caliari MV, Reis ZSN. Association between the chronology of gestation and the morphometrical skin characteristics at childbirth: A development of predictive model. BMJ Health & Care Informatics. 2021;**28**(1):1-8. e100476. DOI: 10.1136/bmjhci-2021-100476

[12] Dhingra S, Asghar A. The epidermal growth pattern in human Fetuses. Indian Journal of Paediatric Dermatology. 2020;**21**(4):287-293. DOI: 10.4103/ijpd.IJPD_42_19

[13] Hoath SB, Maibach HI. Neonatal Skin: Structure and Function. Boca

Raton, Florida, USA: CRC Press; 2003. DOI: 10.1201/b15037

[14] Reis ZSN, Vitral GLN, de Souza IMF, Rego MAS, Guimaraes RN. Newborn skin reflection: Proof of concept for a new approach for predicting gestational age at birth. A cross-sectional study. PLoS One. 2017;**12**(9):e0184734. DOI: 10.1371/journal.pone.0184734

[15] Reis ZSN, Guimarães RN, Rego MAS, de Castro M, Romanelli R, Gaspar JS, et al. Prematurity detection evaluating interaction between the skin of the newborn and light: Protocol for the preemie-test multicentre clinical trial in Brazilian hospitals to validate a new medical device. BMJ Open. 2019;**9**(3):e027442. DOI: 10.2196/16477

[16] Ballard J, Khoury J, Wedig K, Wang L, Eilers-Walsman B, Lipp R. New Ballard score, expanded to include extremely premature infants. The Journal of Pediatrics. 1991;**119**(3):417-423. DOI: 10.1016/s0022-3476(05)82056-6

[17] Capurro H, Konichezky S, Fonseca D, Caldeyro-Barcia R. A simplified method for diagnosis of gestational age in the newborn infant. The Journal of Pediatrics. 1978;**93**(1):120-122. DOI: 10.1016/s0022-3476(78)80621-0

[18] Farr V, Kerridge DF, Mitchell RG. The value of some external characteristics in the assessment of gestational age at birth. Developmental Medicine and Child Neurology. 1966;**8**(6):657-660. DOI: 10.1111/j.1469-8749.1966.tb01823.x

[19] Finnström O. Studies on maturity in newborn infants. IX. Further observations on the use of external characteristics in estimating gestational age. Acta Paediatrica Scandinavica. 1977;**66**(5):601-604. DOI: 10.1111/j.1651-2227.1977.tb07954.x

[20] Fullerton A, Fischer T, Lahti A, Wilhelm KP, Takiwaki H, Serup J. Guidelines for measurement of skin colour and erythema. A report from the standardization Group of the European Society of contact dermatitis. Contact Dermatitis. 1996;**35**(1):1-10. DOI: 10.1111/j.1600-0536.1996.tb02258.x

[21] Stamatas GN, Zmudzka BZ, Kollias N, Beer JZ. Non-invasive measurements of skin pigmentation in situ. Pigment Cell Research. 2004;**17**(6):618-626. DOI: 10.1111/srt.12810

[22] Silva PC, Guimarães RN, Souza RG, Reis ZSN. A quantitative cross-sectional analysis of the melanin index in the skin of preterm newborns and its association with gestational age at birth. Skin Research and Technology. 2020;**26**(3):356-361. DOI: 10.1111/srt.12810

[23] Post PW, Krauss AN, Waldman S, Auld PA. Skin reflectance of newborn infants from 25 to 44 weeks gestational age. Human Biology. 1976;**48**(3):541-557

[24] Reis Z, Vitral G, Guimarães R, Gaspar J, Colosimo E, Taunde S, et al. Premature or small for gestational age discrimination: International Multicenter trial protocol for classification of the low-birth-weight Newborn through the optical properties of the skin. JMIR Research Protocols. 2020;**9**(7):e16477. DOI: 10.2196/16477

[25] Rippon M, Springett K, Walmsley R, Patrick K, Millson S. Ultrasound assessment of skin and wound tissue: Comparison with histology. Skin Research and Technology. 1998;**4**(3):147-154. DOI: 10.1111/j.1600-0846.1998.tb00101.x

[26] Petersen JR, Petersen S, Serup J. High-frequency ultrasound measurement of dermis and subcutaneous fat in

the newborn infant. Skin Research and Technology. 1995;**1**(2):86-89. DOI: 10.1111/j.1600-0846.1995.tb00023.x

[27] Vitral GLN, Aguiar RAPL, de Souza IMF, Rego MAS, Guimarães RN, Reis ZSN. Skin thickness as a potential marker of gestational age at birth despite different fetal growth profiles: A feasibility study. PLoS One. 2018;**13**(4):e0196542. DOI: 10.1371/journal.pone.0196542 A

[28] Kazumi F. Usefulness of comprehensive high - resolution ultrasound imaging in dermatologic field - epidermal cyst. Biomedical Journal of Scientific & Technical Research. 2018;**12**(1):8917-8920. DOI: 10.26717/BJSTR.2018.12.002184

[29] Ashish K, Nelin V, Vitrakoti R, Aryal S, Målqvist M. Validation of the foot length measure as an alternative tool to identify low birth weight and preterm babies in a low-resource setting like Nepal: A cross-sectional study. BMC Pediatrics. 2015;**15**(1):1-8. DOI: 10.1186/s12887-015-0361-4

[30] Srinivasa S, Manasa G, Madhu G. Foot length of newborn: Its correlation with gestational age and various anthropometric parameters. Current Pediatric Research. 2017. Article ID: sea-204690

[31] Wyk LV, Smith J. Postnatal foot length to determine gestational age: A pilot study. Journal of Tropical Pediatrics. 2016;**62**(2):144-151. DOI: 10.1093/tropej/fmv093

[32] Pandey VD, Singh V, Nigam G, Usmani Y, Yadav Y. Fetal foot length for assessment of gestational age: A comprehensive study in North India. Scholars Journal of Applied Medical Sciences. 2015;**3**(1C):139-144. DOI: 10.18203/2320-1770.ijrcog20212972

[33] Stevenson A, Joolay Y, Levetan C, Price C, Tooke L. A comparison of the accuracy of various methods of postnatal gestational age estimation; including Ballard score, foot length, vascularity of the anterior Lens, last menstrual period and also a Clinician's non-structured assessment. Journal of Tropical Pediatrics. 2021;**67**(1):1-12. DOI: 10.1093/tropej/fmaa113

[34] Patel AB, Kulkarni H, Kurhe K, Prakash A, Bhargav S, Parepalli S, et al. Early identification of preterm neonates at birth with a tablet app for the simplified gestational age score (T-SGAS) when ultrasound gestational age dating is unavailable: A validation study. PLoS One. 2020;**15**(8):e0238315. DOI: 10.1371/journal.pone.0238315

[35] McCarton CM, Wallace IF, Divon M, Vaughan HG. Cognitive and neurologic development of the premature, small for gestational age infant through age 6: Comparison by birth weight and gestational age. Pediatrics. 1996;**98** (6 Pt 1):1167-1178

[36] Castro Conde JR, González Campo C, González González NL, Reyes Millán B, González Barrios D, Jiménez Sosa A, et al. Assessment of neonatal EEG background and neurodevelopment in full-term small for their gestational age infants. Pediatric Research. 2020;**88**(1):91-99. DOI: 10.1038/s41390-019-0693-0

[37] World Health Organization. Global Strategy on Digital Health 2020-2025. Geneve: World Health Organization; 2021. Available from: https://www.who.int/docs/default-source/documents/gs4dhdaa2a9f352b0445bafbc79ca799dce4d.pdf. [Accessed: 03-01-2022]

[38] Alliance for Maternal and Newborn Health Improvement (AMANHI)

Gestational Age Study Group. Simplified models to assess newborn gestational age in low-middle income countries: Findings from a multicountry, prospective cohort study. BMJ Global Health. 2021;**6**(9):1-11. e005688. DOI: 10.1136/bmjgh-2021-005688

[39] Rittenhouse KJ, Vwalika B, Keil A, Winston J, Stoner M, Price JT, et al. Improving preterm newborn identification in low-resource settings with machine learning. PLoS One. 2019;**14**(2):e0198919. DOI: 10.1371/journal.pone.0198919

[40] Therrell BL, Padilla CD, Loeber JG, Kneisser I, Saadallah A, Borrajo GJ, et al. Current status of newborn screening worldwide: 2015. Seminars in Perinatology. 2015;**39**(3):171-187. DOI: 10.1053/j.semperi.2015.03.002

[41] Wilson K, Hawken S, Potter BK, Chakraborty P, Walker M, Ducharme R, et al. Accurate prediction of gestational age using newborn screening analyte data. American Journal of Obstetrics and Gynecology. 2016;**214**(4):513.e1-513.e9. DOI: 10.1016/j.ajog.2015.10.017

[42] Wilson K, Hawken S, Murphy MSQ, Atkinson KM, Potter BK, Sprague A, et al. Postnatal prediction of gestational age using Newborn Fetal Hemoglobin levels. eBioMedicine. 2017;**15**:203-209. DOI: 10.1136/bmjopen-2016-015615

[43] Hawken S, Ducharme R, Murphy MSQ, Atkinson KM, Potter BK, Chakraborty P, et al. Performance of a postnatal metabolic gestational age algorithm: A retrospective validation study among ethnic subgroups in Canada. BMJ Open. 2017;7(9):e015615. DOI: 10.1136/bmjopen-2016-015615

[44] Ryckman KK, Berberich SL, Dagle JM. Predicting gestational age using neonatal metabolic markers. American Journal of Obstetrics and Gynecology. 2016;**214**(4):515.e1-515e13. DOI: 10.1016/j.ajog.2015.11.028

[45] Murphy MS, Hawken S, Cheng W, Wilson LA, Lamoureux M, Henderson M, et al. External validation of postnatal gestational age estimation using newborn metabolic profiles in Matlab, Bangladesh. eLife. 2019;**8**:1-15. DOI: 10.7554/eLife.42627

[46] Wilson LA, Murphy MS, Ducharme R, Denize K, Jadavji NM, Potter B, et al. Postnatal gestational age estimation via newborn screening analysis: Application and potential. Expert Review of Proteomics. 2019;**16**(9):727-731. DOI: 10.1136/bmjopen-2016-015615

[47] Hannum G, Guinney J, Zhao L, Zhang L, Hughes G, Sadda S, et al. Genome-wide methylation profiles reveal quantitative views of human aging rates. Molecular Cell. 2013;**49**(2):359-367. DOI: 10.1016/j.molcel.2012.10.016

[48] Knight AK, Craig JM, Theda C, Bækvad-Hansen M, Bybjerg-Grauholm J, Hansen CS, et al. An epigenetic clock for gestational age at birth based on blood methylation data. Genome Biology. 2016;**17**(1):206. DOI: 10.1186/s13059-016-1068-z

[49] Simpkin AJ, Suderman M, Gaunt TR, Lyttleton O, McArdle WL, Ring SM, et al. Longitudinal analysis of DNA methylation associated with birth weight and gestational age. Human Molecular Genetics. 2015;**24**(13):3752-3763. DOI: 10.1093/hmg/ddv119

Chapter 7

Literacy on Skin-to-Skin Contact

María del Carmen Gangotena

Abstract

Strong scientific evidence supports the importance of practicing skin-to-skin contact immediately after childbirth. It is considered a unique time that provides vital advantages and short- and long-term health benefits for infants and mothers. Skin-to-skin contact has proved to enhance social and emotional development and attachment. Other benefits of skin-to-skin contact are the high impact on promoting breastfeeding and healthy eating behaviors. It promotes neurophysiological adjustment to postnatal life. Newborn infants who received SSC cry less, and mothers experience fewer maternal depression symptoms. The newborn infants experienced less pain responding to vitamin K intramuscular injections. This practice has a great value, and it is a natural and instinctive behavior; therefore, it is essential to convey understandable information to pregnant women and their families, permitting them to follow health-informed decisions to support SSC as the best start for their babies.

Keywords: Skin-to-skin contact, breastfeeding, infant health, nutrition, development

1. Introduction

Personal health literacy (PHL) is defined as a person's capacity to procure, understand, and use health information and services needed to make appropriate health decisions and pursue actions for themselves and others [1]. Then, literacy on skin-to-skin contact (SSC) aims to convey understandable information pristinely, providing evidence-based information.

The mother and newborn infant have a physiological need to stay together in SSC, immediately after delivery and in the days and months following birth [2]. SSC is the naked newborn infant's contact with the abdomen or maternal breast without any separation; it is immediate and uninterrupted after birth and should happen for at least sixty minutes without interruptions [3–5].

This chapter presents the relevant scientific evidence on SSC, for a significant impact on health and nutrition during the life of the human being [3, 5].

Current research shows the multiple benefits for both mother and newborn infant [4, 6]. The first hour of life is a particular time called the sensitive period; the newborn baby presents high levels of catecholamines that keep the child in an alert state; meanwhile, the mother's hormonal response of oxytocin and prolactin supports bonding [6, 7]. The practice calms and relaxes both mother and baby, meanwhile regulating the baby's heart rate and breathing, helping them to better adapt to life outside the womb, stimulating digestion and interest in feeding, regulating temperature, enabling the colonization of the baby's skin with the mother's friendly bacteria, thus protecting the baby against infection, and stimulates the release of hormones to support breastfeeding and mothering [7].

In the neonatal unit (NU) improves oxygen saturation, reduces stress levels, particularly following painful procedures, encourages pre-feeding behavior, assists with growth, may reduce hospital stay; improves milk volume if the mother expresses following a period of SSC, with the expressed milk containing the most up-to-date antibodies [6, 7].

In summary, the advantages for a mother's health include the early expulsion of the placenta and reduction of hemorrhage [2, 7]. SSC empowers mothers and enhances parent-infant bonding [4–6, 8–13]. Immediate SSC promotes breastfeeding, increasing successful exclusive breastfeeding [4] and increasing maternal self-efficacy [1–5]. SSC stimulates the eating behaviors of rooting, sucking, and lactating [3]. The advantage for the infant includes decreased stress due to childbirth [6], better thermoregulation, and less crying [6]. Mediated by SSC, the infant acquires a correct grip, feeding sessions are more satisfactory and prolonged, and positive weight gain and development occur. Besides, SSC supports socio-emotional development. Simultaneously, positive feeding behaviors are timely established while improving the newborn infant's digestion [3] and increasing immunity [3]. SSC reduces the risk of infant mortality, nosocomial infections, hyperthermia, and duration of hospital stay [14, 15].

Although SSC is a natural and easy practice to implement, its application still has barriers [3, 16]. The traditional separation between mother and newborn infant is still promoted for evaluations, medical procedures, and other routine processes [3]. It requires a commitment from public health policies and maternal and childcare facilities [16].

SSC literacy should be carried out at all levels, both for maternal and child health personnel and for the community, pregnant women, families, and leaders; SSC may be protected by implementing evidence-based routines at the maternities and hospitals that serve mothers and babies. Therefore, this chapter is essential to promote the advantages of carrying out this beneficial practice from the beginning of life.

2. Definition and history of skin-to-skin contact (SSC)

SSC is defined as the practice where a baby is dried and laid directly on the mother's bare chest after childbirth; meaning that the naked newborn infant is in contact with the abdomen or maternal breast without any separation, both covered in a warm blanket; it is immediate and uninterrupted and for at least an hour or until after the first feed; for at least sixty minutes without interruptions [3, 4, 17]. SSC is a natural and straightforward practice sustained on the need mother, and newborn infant have a physiological and emotional need to stay together in SSC immediately after delivery and in the days and months following birth [2, 17].

In 1978 in Colombia, where preterm infants' mortality reached 70%, early attachment was introduced to alleviate health complications associated with overcrowding, prematurity, nosocomial infections, and the problem of sharing incubators. Dr. Edgar Rey Sanabria, Professor of Neonatology at the National University of Colombia, found that mothers who implemented SSC with low-weight premature infants achieved high rates of exclusive breastfeeding, lowered infant mortality, and decreased the time of internment; also, infant mortality decreased from 70% to 30% [3].

3. Skin-to-skin contact and breastfeeding and eating behaviors

SSC supports socio-emotional development. Relevant scientific evidence on SSC shows a high impact on promoting breastfeeding [3, 5, 17]; SSC stimulates the eating behaviors of rooting, sucking, and lactating [3]. Mediated by SSC, the infant acquires a correct grip, feeding sessions are more satisfactory and prolonged, and positive weight gain and development occur. Simultaneously, positive feeding behaviors are established timely while improving the newborn infant's digestion [3] and increasing immunity [3].

The evidence shows that SSC is an accessible practice promoting breastfeeding during the neonatal period [2, 5, 18], protecting against infections and future allergies [16, 19]. Breastfeeding promotes increased blood circulation and temperature in the breast area, promoting breast milk production and helping keep the newborn infant warm [3, 5].

SSC and immediate breastfeeding are closely related and mutually beneficial [3, 5, 20]. Newborn infants' SSC is related to the timely initiation of breastfeeding [2, 17, 21] within the first hour of life, becoming a fundamental practice for child survival and proper development [3, 16, 19]. This protective benefit extends to six months of age.

UNICEF recommends that breastfeeding begins within the first hour of life, continues exclusively for the first six months of life, and continues with healthy and adequate complementary foods until the infant is two years old [16, 19]. SSC allows the infant to stand firmly against the mother's breast, often between her breasts, with the mother in a semi-reclined, supported position [3, 9]. Preterm infants can latch onto the breast and suck from week 27 of gestation; as soon as they are stable, they can begin breastfeeding [3, 9]. SSC facilitates a transition to exclusive breastfeeding [3, 5, 9].

SSC beyond childbirth can facilitate the duration of breastfeeding. SSC enhances positive maternal interactions at one week, two months, and three months after delivery, supporting mothers' decision to practice breastfeeding [22].

4. Skin-to-skin contact and early adjustments to life

SSC promotes neurophysiological adjustment to postnatal life [3, 4, 19]. It helps achieve stability while transitioning from uterine life to living outside of the womb [3]. SSC helps populate the newborn infant's microbiome while preventing hypothermia because it regulates the newborn infant's body temperature while stabilizing the cardio-respiratory system and regulating blood glucose [3, 5]. SSC has a positive stimulus on a newborn infant's digestion because it promotes colonization from the mother's beneficial bacteria [5]

5. Skin-to-skin contact and psychosocial health and development

After birth, the newborn infant experiences a sensitive period that enhances positive behaviors development beyond the first day of life [2, 5, 18]. Furthermore, researchers found that SSC promotes psychosocial health, increasing the infant's perception as an active agent in social interactions in her surrounding space [18].

In a longitudinal study, they found that SSC during the postpartum period has long-term benefits for child development. Premature infants who received SSC during the first weeks of age, at age ten [10] showed reduced stress response, improved mature autonomic functioning, organized sleep, better cognitive control, and better mother-child interaction [23].

A twenty-year longitudinal study indicates that Kangaroo Mother Care (KMC) had significant, long-lasting social and behavioral protective effects 20 years after the intervention [24].

6. Skin-to-skin contact and psychosocial health and parents' anxiety and depression

Newborn infants who received SSC cry less after the first hour of life [3, 5], and mothers and infants experience and exhibit more relaxed behaviors [2, 3, 5, 18]. Mothers experience fewer maternal depression symptoms and postpartum stress [25, 26]. Also, the newborn infant can reach states of calm more quickly because they recover faster from the stress caused by birth, as evidenced by measuring cortisol's blood levels [2, 17].

SSC generates feelings of attachment between the mother and her newborn infant, allowing them to recognize each other and respond to the infant's needs in a timely and secure manner [5, 18]. Parents who have practiced SSC also feel more confident in caring for their infants [4, 5]. Besides, parents develop strong feelings toward the newborn infant and feel more security and less anxiety [3, 5, 8, 25].

The enhanced interaction results in more positive interactions, increasing the mother's satisfaction in the postpartum period, which contributes to a better relationship and successful breastfeeding [2, 5, 20, 21]. Practicing SSC, the mother suffers a decrease in uterine bleeding, and her chances of suffering a postpartum hemorrhage decrease [16, 19]. Mothers release hormones, oxytocin and endorphins, which positively reduce postpartum uterine bleeding [3, 5]. Newborn infants, who experienced SSC, suck efficiently, contributing to a woman's breast health [16, 19]. The physiological hormonal effect includes positive maternal feelings, calmness, and anxiety reduction [5, 21].

In cesarian section cases, where the mother's health is unstable and caring for preterm and underweight infants, the father can also provide SSC. These two scenarios empower the father to assist with the newborn infant's care, creating trust and attachment [3, 8]. The father warms the infant in these circumstances because his chest temperature does not fluctuate [3], as in postpartum women. Infants who were attached to their fathers cry significantly less and sleep soundly. Infants can immediately transition to SSC with their mother and begin breastfeeding [3]. From fathers' SSC, newborn infants benefit by stabilizing body temperature and improving cardio-respiratory function and glucose levels [3, 5]. Fathers who experienced SSC experienced greater feelings of attachment and feelings of closeness to their newborn infants [3, 8].

SSC stimulates the release of oxytocin (OT), decreasing infant salivary cortisol (SC) levels. Facilitation of SSC may be an effective intervention to reduce parent and infant stress in the neonatal intensive care units (NICU), promoting responsiveness and synchrony in parent-infant interactions [27].

7. Skin-to-skin contact and cesarian section, preterm and premature newborn infants

The protocols promote the mother and her newborn infant's separation in cesarian delivery, an essential barrier for SSC. It is not promoted that the father practices SSC if the woman cannot achieve it. Positive action is to spread the benefits that entail this natural and simple practice, both at the individual and community level and to support SSC at the public health policy level [3, 16, 19].

Scientific evidence shows that, in intensive care units. SSC in stable infants improves physiological stability, growth, and weight gain and reduces the need to supply oxygen externally [3], acquiring stability in cardio-respiratory function [2, 17].

SSC benefits to preterm and premature newborn infants have been demonstrated widely by the Kangaroo Mother Program (KMP) [2], an early, continuous, and prolonged SSC between mother and newborn infant. It should be started as soon as the infant presents an absence of severe apnea, desaturation, and bradycardia [3]. KMP has shown benefits for infant survival, bodily regulation, and successful breastfeeding initiation [16, 21].

Furthermore, preterm and underweight infants who experience SSC are discharged in fewer days. If infants receive SSC, their system is colonized with normal maternal flora, promoting a strengthened immune system [3]. SSC protects infants from prevalent infections in care units and predisposing allergens [3]. Furthermore, infants who received skin-to-skin contact were discharged faster than those who did not [3].

8. Skin-to-skin contact and procedural pain

Preterm infants (PTI) who received SSC had markedly reduced procedural pain (5; 28-31) on the scale when heel pricks were experienced [28, 29]. SSC reduces procedural pain in newborn infants [30–32] and significantly reduces the duration of crying by releasing oxytocin [3, 5, 29]. Oxytocin, becoming a natural analgesic, the cry lasts less, and the infant comes to a calm and relaxed state sooner [3, 28, 31, 33].

A Cochrane meta-analysis showed that infants in skin-to-skin contact during intra-muscular injection (IM) were more prone to low pain after IM and during pain recovery; based on cut-off scores for the Neonatal Infant Pain Scale (NPS). Most infants can be expected to experience a reduction in pain related to at least ten [10] minutes of the duration of SSC before the painful procedure is effective for PTI experiencing heel pricks and for term infants (TI) receiving (IM) injection [31].

The newborn infants that received Kangaroo Care (KC) experienced less pain responding to vitamin K intramuscular (IM) injections, and the duration of crying was less than newborn infants that did not receive KC [34].

C-section newborn infants who received SSC showed a significantly lower score on the Neonatal Infant Pain Scale (NIPS), responding to vitamin K injection administered sixty minutes after birth [32]. Besides, mothers experienced an increased satisfaction rate regarding their childbirth experience [32].

PTI born thirty [33] weeks gestational age or older showed a statistically significant reduction of pain, assessed using facial action (NFCS), sleep-wake (Behavioral state), infant cry and heart rate (HR), during the puncture, heel squeeze, and the post phases of heel prick when experiencing SSC fifteen [15] minutes before, during, and after the procedure [35].

The heart rate (HR) of preterm newborn infants that received heel Stick was significantly minor in those who received KC for thirty [33] and fifteen [15] minutes, as well as their recovery, was shorter, revealing a significant effect on reducing autonomic pain response in PTI [33].

PTI during a blood sampling procedure with venepuncture showed a significantly smaller increase in oxygenated hemoglobin when lying in their mothers' chest in SSC, compared to those laying in their incubator or crib [31].

9. Literacy on the nine developmental stages of the newborn infant

Health staff working in maternities and MCH facilities should receive training to fully understand the newborn infant's instinctive behavior while SSC during the first hour of life of the healthy alert newborn infant [6]. The mother and the family should receive education on the newborn infants' behaviors on SSC during the antenatal encounters with MCH staff [6]. Widström and colleagues found that the parents aware of the nine stages respond positively and identify the newborn infant's actions [6].

SSC supports the baby's journey through the nine instinctive stages—birth cry, relaxation, awakening, activity, rest, crawling, familiarization, suckling, and sleeping. The sensitized family and health staff will guard the newborn infant's behavior of SSC and the nine stages, acknowledging that the mother and her baby must stay together for the first hours of life [6]. Besides, the evidence shows that interrupting the natural stream of the nine stages and SSC is related to fewer rates of early breastfeeding [2, 17, 21, 36].

After Childbirth, stage 1 is initiated, called birth crying, and it is when the babies' lungs expand for the first time, and the newborn infant starts to breathe, clearing the aerial ways. The baby is on keen alert and should be placed in a semi-prone mother's chest where the newborn infant leads to stabilize the breathing rate [5]. Besides, the mothers' confidence grows when she has the baby in her chest [2, 19, 20, 23, 26].

Stage 2 is called relaxation; the newborn infant stays quietly and relaxes over the mothers' chest, listening to her heartbeat. During stage 2, it is recommended to apply the APGAR assessment and the IM and other procedures [10]. It is essential to leave the baby without interrupting [5].

Following is stage 3, awakening means the transition from relaxation to activity. During this stage, the baby does tiny movements of the head, arms, and fingers; the newborn moves the mouth, opens the eyes, and blinks [4, 5].

Stage 4 is activity; the baby moves the upper part of the body; the newborn's head may be lifted to search for the mother's chest. The baby's limbs expand to reach the woman's breast; rooting is evident during the activity stage. In preparation for breastfeeding, the newborn moved the tongue; the evidence links the secretions of the Montgomery glands with the baby's behavioral responses [4–6]. The newborn touches the nipple and receives the taste through hand-to-breast movements, stimulating the rooting and crawling movements to reach the breast [4–6, 37, 38]. It is not recommended to interfere with the sensory olfactory connection between the newborn and her mother [39]. Furthermore, the fetus learned to recognize the mother's voice; now, the mother should talk to the newborn to cause eye contact in the first half-hour of life, promoting bonding between them [6, 36, 40].

Stage 5, called resting and may be present in the other stages, the newborn may require resting at any other stage, health staff and parents must respect the baby's rhythm not interrupting SSC and separating the infant from the mother's touch [4–6].

Stage 6 is crawling; the baby moves from the chest to the nipple; during this stage, the infant exercises the stepping reflex, contributing to the contractions in the uterus, helping to expel the placenta and decrease hemorrhage [4–6]. It is helpful to place a supportive pillow or towel to protect the newborn efforts to reach the nipple, and it is necessary; the mother may support the baby by putting her palm under the newborn foot [6].

Stage 7 is called familiarization; the newborn is gaining confidence; the mother should respond to the calls the baby is making while approaching the nipple and licking it. There should not be interrupting or rushing; the 7th stage can be 20 minutes or longer [6]. Besides, the rooting reflex and the infant's tongue coordination increase, preparing the baby to start suckling the colostrum [6].

Stage 8 is suckling; the infant attaches to the mother's nipple and starts breastfeeding. The baby should widely open the mouth to the entire areola [2–5], protecting against damage to the nipple. When suckling starts, the newborn is wholly focused on the task; the health staff does not need to help the newborn to attach to the mother's breast; the evidence is clear about the importance to start breastfeeding during the first hour of life to promote successful breastfeeding [2–7].

Stage 9 is sleeping; the newborn finishes to suckle in at least one hour after birth, becoming quiet and subsequently falling asleep. The OT promotes releasing gastrointestinal hormones (GIH), such as cholecystokinin (CKK) and gastrin [2–6]. The high levels of CKK cause a relaxing postprandial sleep in both the baby and the mother [6].

During the nine stages, health staff must accompany the mother and the baby through keen observation of the newborn health status and breathing functions.

10. Barriers to skin-to-skin contact

Although SSC is a natural and easy practice to implement, its application still has barriers [2, 3, 16]. It requires a commitment from public health policies and maternal and childcare facilities [16]. The traditional separation between mother and newborn infant is still promoted for evaluations, medical procedures, and other routine processes [3].

Sometimes health staff does not recognize the importance of SSC and its implications for the infant and his family [16, 19]. They may be resistant to change, and it is essential to promote awareness and perform routine training [16, 19, 41]. Some parents' beliefs about keeping the newborn infant warm and the importance of remaining in an incubator are a barrier to SSC [37]. In other cases, family visits do not allow parents' privacy to experience SSC with their newborn infants [37, 38]. Additionally, crowded maternities can also be uncomfortable for the mother, the father, and the newborn infant [38, 41].

11. Conclusions

Undoubtedly, skin-to-skin contact has robust evidence that supports the importance to introduce the practice immediately after childbirth. It is considered a unique time to enhance the bonding between the newborn infant and the mother; besides providing vital advantages and short- and long-term health benefits for infants and mothers.

It is imperative to improve the understanding of SSC as a great value and a need for the newborn infant and the mother. SSC is a natural and instinctive behavior; therefore, it is indispensable to present the scientific evidence in an organized, understandable, and evidence-based manner to support maternal and child health professionals who wish to implement the practice in hospitals and maternal and child centers. Nevertheless, the friendly information must be available for pregnant women and their families, permitting them to follow health-informed decisions to support SSC as the best start for their babies.

Promoting skin-to-skin contact between the baby and the mother is a unique experience with profound benefits for families and communities. It is valuable for health staff at maternity units and parents to understand the nine stages of infant behavioral development in the first hour of life; it is a sensitive period that promotes bonding and early attachment.

Conflict of interest

"The authors declare no conflict of interest."

Acronyms and abbreviations

PHL	personal health literacy
SSC	skin-to-skin contact
KMC	Kangaroo Mother Care
UNICEF	United Nations Infant and Children's Fund
OT	oxytocin
SC	salivary cortisol
NICU	neonatal intensive care units
KMP	Kangaroo Mother Program
PTI	preterm infants
TI	term infants
NPS	Neonatal Infant Pain Scale
NFCS	neonatal facial action
HR	heart rate

Author details

María del Carmen Gangotena
St. Francis Xavier University, Antigonish, NS, Canada

*Address all correspondence to: x2017wvd@stfx.ca

References

[1] Santana S, Brach C, Harris L, Ochiai E, Blakey C, Bevington F, et al. Updating health literacy for Healthy People 2030: Defining its importance for a new decade in public health: Defining its importance for a new decade in public health. Journal of Public Health Management Practice. 2021;**27**(Suppl. 6): S258-S264

[2] Aghdas K, Talat K, Sepideh B. Effect of immediate and continuous mother-infant skin-to-skin contact on breastfeeding self-efficacy of primiparous women: a randomised control trial. Women and Birth. 2014;**27**(1):37-40

[3] Sheryl Meyers BS. Skin-to-skin contact. Journal of Alternative Medicine Research. 1 Jul 2015;**7**(3):185

[4] Crenshaw JT. Healthy birth practice #6: Keep mother and newborn together-it's best for mother, newborn, and breastfeeding. Journal of Perinatal Education. 2019;**28**(2):108-115

[5] Moore ER, Bergman N, Anderson GC, Medley N. Early skin-to-skin contact for mothers and their healthy newborn infants. Cochrane Database System Review. 2016;**11**(11):CD003519

[6] Widström A-M, Brimdyr K, Svensson K, Cadwell K, Nissen E. Skin-to-skin contact the first hour after birth, underlying implications and clinical practice. Acta Paediatric. 2019;**108**(7):1192-1204

[7] Safari K, Saeed AA, Hasan SS, Moghaddam-Banaem L. The effect of mother and newborn early skin-to-skin contact on initiation of breastfeeding, newborn temperature and duration of third stage of labor. International Breastfeed Journal. Dec 2018;**13**(1):1-8

[8] Varela N, Tessier R, Tarabulsy G, Pierce T. Cortisol and blood pressure levels decreased in fathers during the first hour of skin-to-skin contact with their premature babies. Acta Paediatric. 2018;**107**(4):628-632

[9] Campbell-Yeo ML, Disher TC, Benoit BL, Johnston CC. Understanding kangaroo care and its benefits to preterm infants. Pediatric Health, Medicine and Therapeutics. 2015;**6**:15

[10] Blomqvist YT, Ewald U, Gradin M, Nyqvist KH, Rubertsson C. Initiation and extent of skin-to-skin care at two Swedish neonatal intensive care units. Acta Paediatric. 2013;**102**(1):22-28

[11] Finigan V, Long T. Skin-to-skin contact: multicultural perspectives on birth fluids and birth "dirt": Cultural perspectives on birth fluids. International Nursing Review. 2014;**61**(2):270-277

[12] Kymre IG, Bondas T. Balancing preterm infants' developmental needs with parents' readiness for skin-to-skin care: a phenomenological study. International Journal of Quality Studies and Health Well-being. 2013;**8**(1):21370

[13] Mazúchová L, Kelčíková S, Maskalová E, Malinovská N, Grendár M. Mother-infant bonding and its associated factors during postpartum period. Kontakt. 2021;**23**(2):126-132

[14] Conde-Agudelo A, Díaz-Rossello JL. Kangaroo mother care to reduce morbidity and mortality in low birthweight infants. Cochrane Database System Review. 2016;**2017**(8):CD002771

[15] Goudard MJ, Lamy ZC, Marba ST, Cavalcante MC, Dos Santos AM, Vivian MD, et al. Skin-to-skin contact

and deaths in newborns weighing up to 1800 grams: a cohort study. Jornal de Pediatria. 17 Oct 2021

[16] Implementation guidance: protecting, promoting, and supporting breastfeeding in facilities providing maternity and newborn services: the revised Baby-friendly Hospital Initiative 2018 [Internet]. Who.int. [cited 2022 Feb 11]. Available from: https://www.who.int/publications-detail-redirect/9789241513807

[17] Skin-to-skin contact [Internet]. Baby Friendly Initiative. 2017 [cited 2022 Feb 18]. Available from: https://www.unicef.org.uk/babyfriendly/baby-friendly-resources/implementing-standards-resources/skin-to-skin-contact/

[18] Ruxer DJ, Brewer T, Mateer K, Burkhardt M, Shay M. The impact of increased skin-to-skin contact with the mother in breastfeeding neonates on exclusive breastfeeding at 4 and 8 weeks postpartum. Clinical Lactation (Amarillo). 2015;**6**(2):75-80

[19] Bigelow AE, Power M. The effect of mother-infant skin-to-skin contact on infants' response to the Still Face Task from newborn to three months of age. Infant Behavior Develpment. 2012;**35**(2):240-251

[20] Bigelow AE, Power M, Gillis DE, Maclellan-Peters J, Alex M, McDonald C. Breastfeeding, skin-to-skin contact, and mother-infant interactions over infants' first three months: Breastfeeding, skin-to-skin, maternal interactions. Infant Mental Health Journal. 2014;**35**(1):51-62

[21] Nutrition, Food Safety. Implementation guidance: protecting, promoting, and supporting breastfeeding in facilities providing maternity and newborn services: the revised Baby-friendly Hospital Initiative 2018 [Internet]. Who.int. World Health Organization; 2018. [cited 2022 Feb 11]. Available from: https://www.who.int/publications/i/item/9789241513807

[22] Mellin PS, Poplawski DT, DeFreest N, Massler K, Gole A. Does skin-to-skin contact at birth really make a difference in exclusive breastfeeding rates at discharge? Journal of Obstetric, Gynecologic, and Neonatal Nursing. 2012;**41**:S141-S142

[23] Alex MR, MacLellan-Peters J. The relationship among skin-to-skin contact, breastfeeding, and mother–infant interaction: Implications for nursing. Journal of Obstetric, Gynecologic, and Neonatal Nursing. 2013;**42**:S88-S89

[24] Feldman R, Rosenthal Z, Eidelman AI. Maternal-preterm skin-to-skin contact enhances child physiologic organization and cognitive control across the first 10 years of life. Biological Psychiatry. 2014;**75**(1):56-64

[25] Charpak N, Tessier R, Ruiz JG, Hernandez JT, Uriza F, Villegas J, et al. Twenty-year follow-up of kangaroo mother care versus traditional care. Pediatrics. 2017;**139**(1):e20162063

[26] Bigelow A, Power M, MacLellan-Peters J, Alex M, McDonald C. Effect of mother/infant skin-to-skin contact on postpartum depressive symptoms and maternal physiological stress. Journal of Obstetric, Gynecologic, and Neonatal Nursing. 2012;**41**(3):369-382

[27] Zauderer C, Goldman S. Cesarean mothers' perception of benefits associated with skin-to-skin contact. Journal of Obstetric, Gynecologic, and Neonatal Nursing. 2012;**41**:S150-S151

[28] Cong X, Cusson RM, Walsh S, Hussain N, Ludington-Hoe SM,

Zhang D. Effects of skin-to-skin contact on autonomic pain responses in preterm infants. Journal of Pain. 2012;**13**(7):636-645

[29] Castral TC, Warnock F, Leite AM, Haas VJ, Scochi CGS. The effects of skin-to-skin contact during acute pain in preterm newborns. European Journal of Pain. 2008;**12**(4):464-471

[30] Vittner D, McGrath J, Robinson J, Lawhon G, Cusson R, Eisenfeld L, et al. Increase in oxytocin from skin-to-skin contact enhances development of parent-infant relationship. Biological Research Nursing. 2018;**20**(1):54-62

[31] Disher T, Benoit B, Johnston C, Campbell-Yeo M. Skin-to-skin contact for procedural pain in neonates: acceptability of novel systematic review synthesis methods and GRADEing of the evidence. Journal of Advanced Nursing. 2017;**73**(2):504-519

[32] Johnston C, Campbell-Yeo M, Disher T, Benoit B, Fernandes A, Streiner D, et al. Skin-to-skin care for procedural pain in neonates. Cochrane Database System Review. 2017;**2**(2):CD008435

[33] Olsson E, Ahlsén G, Eriksson M. Skin-to-skin contact reduces near-infrared spectroscopy pain responses in premature infants during blood sampling. Acta Paediatric. 2016;**105**(4):376-380

[34] Pasquier J-C, Blouin S, Daigle K, Corriveau S, Thibodeau D, Goffaux P. Immediate skin-to-skin contact after caesarean delivery to improve neonatal pain tolerance. American Journal of Obstetrics and Gynecology. 2013;**208**(1):S322

[35] Abeling BA, Thacker AD. The impact of kangaroo care on pain in term newborns receiving intramuscular injections. Journal of Obstetric, Gynecologic, & Neonatal Nursings. 2013;**42**:S89

[36] Anderzen-Carlsson A, Lamy ZC, Eriksson M. Parental experiences of providing skin-to-skin care to their newborn infant—Part 1: A qualitative systematic review. International Journal of Qualitative Studies on Health and Well-Being. 2014;**9**:24906

[37] Mörelius E, Anderson GC. Neonatal nurses' beliefs about almost continuous parent-infant skin-to-skin contact in neonatal intensive care. Journal of Clinical Nursing. 2015;**24**(17-18):2620-2627

[38] Koopman I, Callaghan-Koru JA, Alaofin O, Argani CH, Farzin A. Early skin-to-skin contact for healthy full-term infants after vaginal and caesarean delivery: A qualitative study on clinician perspectives. Journal of Clinical Nursing. 2016;**25**(9-10):1367-1376

[39] Ferrarello D, Hatfield L. Barriers to skin-to-skin care during the postpartum stay. MCN: The American Journal of Maternal/Child Nursing. 2014;**39**(1):56-61

[40] Essa RM, Ismail NI. Effect of early maternal/newborn skin-to-skin contact after birth on the duration of third stage of labor and initiation of breastfeeding. Journal of Nursing Education and Practice. 2 Feb 2015;**5**(4):98

[41] Castral TC, Warnock F, Leite AM, Haas VJ, Scochi CGS. The effects of skin-to-skin contact during acute pain in preterm newborns. Acute Pain. 2008;**10**(2):108-109

Section 5

Contraception

Chapter 8

Utilization of Implant Contraceptive Methods and Associated Factors among Reproductive-Age Women in Ethiopia

Birye Dessalegn Mekonnen and Chalachew Adugna Wubneh

Abstract

Implants are more effective, enable women to control their reproductive lives better, and are better options of contraception than other long-term family planning methods. Researches are required to provide up-to-date evidence for policymakers, and other stakeholders working on the family planning program in Ethiopia as the evidence from different studies conducted in Ethiopia on implants contraceptive method utilization was highly varied and not conclusive. Therefore, the current study aims to determine the magnitude of implant contraceptive utilization and its associated factors among reproductive-age women in Ethiopia. A population-based cross-sectional study has conducted using secondary data analysis from the EDHS 2016. A total of 14,593 reproductive-age women participated in this study. The analysis was performed using the SPSS version 20 statistical package. Bivariate and multivariable logistic regression analysis was performed to identify independent predictors of implant contraceptive methods utilization. Statistical significance was declared at p-value <0.05. The prevalence of implant contraceptive utilization among reproductive-age women in Ethiopia was 9.4% (95% CI: 8.8, 10.0). The results of multivariable logistic regression showed that marital status, place of residence, number of living children, history of a terminated pregnancy, husband desire for more children, decision making on contraceptive use, knowledge on contraceptives, discussed FP with the healthcare worker and heard family planning message on television were independent predictors of implants contraceptive use among reproductive-age women in Ethiopia. The study showed that the magnitude of implant contraceptive utilization among reproductive-age women in Ethiopia is very low as compared with the national 2020 plan. The finding of this study suggests any intervention strategy which is designed and being implemented to promote implants contraceptive method utilization should consider the aforementioned factors for its better success. Besides, the provision of quality counseling and information on FP, and women empowerment should be promoted so that women can freely decide on the type of contraceptive they would like to use. Moreover, emphasis should be given to rural women and no television access to implants contraceptive method utilization.

Keywords: implant contraceptive methods, reproductive age women, EDHS 2016, Ethiopia

1. Introduction

Population growth becomes an urgent global concern with an expected half of the world's population growth will be concentrated in just nine countries [1]. With the highest rate of population growth, Africa is expected to account for more than half of the world population growth between 2015 and 2050 [2]. Ethiopia is among countries with higher fertility rates in the world and high populous nations in Africa [3]. Fertility rates are determinant actors of the human development index (HDI) affecting life expectancy, education, per capita income, and other indicators [4]. The role of family planning (FP) in decreasing fertility rate which could reduce maternal and child mortality, and other health costs thereby improving maternal and child health is widely advocated [5, 6].

Implants such as Implanon, Sino implant, and Jadelle are among the modern contraceptive methods that are long-acting, reversible, and hormonal contraceptives [7, 8]. Contraceptive implants are one of the most effective family planning methods which widely available and have increased global acceptance [9, 10]. Implants are better options of contraception than other long-term family planning methods as they easily insert and remove and have fewer side effects [10].

The high rate of implants utilization by couples is indicative of FP program effectiveness within a country in addition to couples' success in spacing and limiting their births [11]. Also, implants play a crucial role in the prevention of unintended pregnancies and abortions as well as in the reduction of maternal mortality and morbidity related to complications of pregnancy and childbirth [12]. Furthermore, the use of implants is comparatively the preferred method of contraception than injectable contraceptives which should be taken every 3 months and daily pills as implants are effective from 3 to 5 years in preventing pregnancy as well as rapid return to usual fertility as soon as implants are removed [10]. However, an analysis of Demographic and Health Surveys (DHS) from four Sub- Saharan Africa (SSA) countries revealed that the proportion of women who utilized implants was much lower than short-acting methods [13].

Though implant acceptance is at an increasing rate, of reproductive-age women who used contraceptive methods, only 0.3% globally, and 7% in Africa utilized implants [9, 14]. Furthermore, in many SSA countries, less than 5% of reproductive-age women are using long-acting contraceptives [15].

In Ethiopia, the ministry of health has planned to increase contraceptive implants to 33% in the method mix in 2015 [16]. However, the Ethiopian demographic and health survey (EDHS) of 2016 showed that only 8% of women utilized implants which indicated that the plan was not achieved [3]. To increase the level of implants utilization among women in Ethiopia, different strategies have been introduced such as practicing community level implants insertion by trained health extension workers (HEWs), and provision of contraceptives implants with free cost as of other contraceptives at all levels of health care [13, 17]. Still, short-acting methods are the dominant contraceptives in the current contraceptive method mix of the country [3, 18].

Studies have been done to determine the prevalence of implant utilization and to identify factors that contribute to the low utilization of implants in Ethiopia [7–9, 15, 19]. Evidence from the abovementioned studies conducted in Ethiopia was highly varied and the results are inconsistent. More research therefore required to provide up-to-date evidence for policymakers, programmers, and other stakeholders working on FP in Ethiopia to solve problems related to implants contraceptive utilization based on evidence. Therefore, the current study aims to assess the magnitude of implant contraceptive utilization and its associated factors among reproductive-age women in Ethiopia based on all-inclusive 2016 EDHS data.

2. Methods

2.1 Study design and period

A nationwide population-based cross-sectional study was conducted using secondary data analysis from the EDHS 2016. The survey data collection was carried out from January 18, 2016, to June 27, 2016.

2.2 Data source and population

The data used for the current study was extracted from 2016 EDHS which was stratified into urban and rural areas. The EDHS data collection procedure followed a two-stage sampling technique to select representative respondents of independent enumeration areas in each stratum. A total of 645 clusters (202 in urban and 443 in rural) enumeration areas were selected using probability proportional allocation to the size of enumeration area in the first stage while 28 households per cluster with an equal probability systematic selection were selected from the newly formed household list in the second stage. Consecutively, a total of 18,008 households were selected for the 2016 EDHS out of which 16,650 households were identified and interviewed yielding a response rate of 92.5%. From 16,650 interviewed households, 15,683 were reproductive age women and completed the interview making a response rate of 94.2% [3]. Finally, women who were reported to be pregnant at the time of the survey were excluded, and data were weighted to adjust for non-response and differences in the probability of selection. Thus, the analysis for this study was restricted to the 14,593 (weighted) reproductive-age women who met the eligibility criteria. Women's questionnaire which contains five different parts including the FP component was used to collect information.

2.3 Variables of the study

Outcome variable: The outcome variable for this study was the utilization of implants which was categorized into two outcome categories: the 'user of implants' women who was using either Implanon or Sino Implant or Jadelle user during EDHS data collection period) and 'non-user of implants' (women who were not using either Implanon or Sino Implant or Jadelle user during EDHS data collection period).

Independent variables: The independent variables were grouped into three categories to see their influence on implant contraceptive use. These included socio-demographic variables (age of the woman, educational status, place of residence, current working status, and wealth index), reproductive and fertility decision making related variables (age at first sex, age at first childbirth, history of abortion, number of living children, fertility preference, husband's desire for more children, the decision on contraceptive use) and exposure to mass media and family planning messages variables (heard family planning messages on radio, heard family planning messages on TV, heard family planning messages on newspapers, visited by a health worker, health worker talked about family planning, visited health facility and told about family planning in the health facility) and women's knowledge on any contraceptives.

3. Statistical analysis

After getting permission, the data was downloaded from the MEASURE DHS database: https://www.dhsprogram.com/data/dataset_admin/login_main.cfm. Statistical package for social science (SPSS) version 20 was used for statistical analysis. Descriptive analysis was used to summarize the distribution of selected background characteristics of the study participants. Frequency tables and graphs were used to summarize and present findings. The data were weighted to adjust for non-response and account for the disproportionate sampling. Bivariate logistic regression analysis was used to select variables fitted for multivariable logistic regression. Variables with a p-value of less than 0.2 in the bivariate logistic regression were included in the multivariable logistic regression. Before running the final model, multicollinearity between candidate variables was checked using variance inflation factor (VIF). Multivariable logistic regression analysis was performed to identify independent predictors of implant contraceptive methods utilization among reproductive-age women in Ethiopia. Adjusted odds ratio (AOR) and 95% confidence interval (CI) were respectively calculated to measure the association between predictor variables and implant contraceptive utilization. Results were considered statistically significant for p-values <0.05. finally, model fitness was checked using Hosmer and Lemeshow's test.

4. Results

4.1 Socio-demographic and socio-economic characteristics of women

The study result was analyzed based on 14,593 reproductive age women in the 2016 EDHS dataset. The mean age of women was 27.1 (± 8.11) years with the majority (24.8%) of women were aged 15–19 years. The majority, 11,468 (78.6%) of women were married, and 9707 (66.5%) were Orthodox religious followers. Out of reproductive age women interviewed, 1760 (12.1%) were from the Oromia region. Concerning the residence of participants, 10,613 (72.7%) were rural residents. About, 9559 (65.5%) of women were not working at the time of the survey. Regarding educational status, 6880 (47.1%) were not educated and 4662 (31.9%) women had completed primary education. About, 4713 (32.3%) of the women were from the poorest family (**Table 1**).

4.2 Reproductive and obstetric characteristics of women

More than three out of five (61.8%) reproductive-age women have started their first sex before the age of 18 years with the mean age of 17.1 (SD ± 5.58) years. The mean age of first childbirth for those who gave birth was 24.88 (SD ± 4.64) years with about half (50.1%) of women giving birth in their age of 18–24 years. The mean number of living children was 2.0 (SD ± 1.8) with more than two-fifths (42.6%)

Variables	Frequency	Percent
Age		
15–19	3612	24.8
20–24	2277	15.6
25–29	2885	19.8
30–34	2626	18.0
35–39	1997	13.7
40–44	833	5.7
45–49	363	2.5
Marital status		
Married	11,468	78.6
Never married/divorced/widowed/separated	3125	21.4
Religion		
Orthodox	9707	66.5
Muslim	4194	28.7
Protestant	504	3.5
Catholic	188	1.3
Place of residence		
Urban	3980	27.3
Rural	10,613	72.7
Educational level		
No formal education	6880	47.1
Primary school	4662	31.9
Secondary school	1965	13.5
Higher education	1086	7.5
Respondents' current working status		
Yes	5034	34.5
No	9559	65.5
Monthly income		
Poorest	4713	32.3
Poorer	2611	17.9
Middle	2594	17.8
Richer	2389	16.4
Richest	2286	15.6
Region		
Tigray	1297	8.9
Afar	1365	9.4
Amhara	1309	9.0
Oromia	1760	12.1
Somalia	1592	10.9
Benishangul	1027	7.0
SNNPR	1659	11.4
Gambela	1017	7.0
Harari	895	6.1
Dire Dawa	1089	7.4
Addis Ababa	1583	10.8

Table 1.
Socio-demographic and socio-economic characteristics of reproductive age women in Ethiopia, 2016.

of women having 1–2 living children. Only, 1107 (7.6%) of women had a history of terminated pregnancy. Around, 4961 (34%) of the women want to have children after 2 years. Concerning partners' desire to have children, 9494 (65.1%) reported that their husbands need to have more children. Regarding decision-making on

Variables	Frequency	Percent
Age at first sex		
Less than 18 years	9024	61.8
18–24 years	5143	35.1
25 and above years	426	2.9
Age at first childbirth		
Not had childbirth	318	2.2
Less than 18 years	5737	39.3
18–24 years	7319	50.1
25 and above years	1219	8.4
Number of living children (parity)		
None	4440	30.4
1 to 2	6216	42.6
3 to 4	3133	21.5
5 and more	804	5.5
Does husband want to have an additional child?		
Yes	9494	65.1
No	5099	34.9
History of a terminated pregnancy		
Yes	1107	7.6
No	13,486	92.4
Fertility preference		
Wants within 2 years	3714	25.5
Wants after 2 years	4961	34.0
Wants no more children	2785	19.1
Undecided	3133	21.4
Decision maker for using contraception		
Mainly respondent	2247	15.4
Mainly husband/partner	8355	57.3
Jointly	3079	21.1
Others	912	6.2

Table 2.
Reproductive and obstetric characteristics of reproductive age women in Ethiopia, 2016.

contraceptive use, 3079 (21.1%) reproductive age women made the decision jointly with their husbands (**Table 2**).

4.3 Exposure to mass media and family planning messages

About three-fourths, 10,978 (75.2%) of women did not hear family planning messages on the radio for the last few months. The majority, 13,666 (93.6%) of women did not hear family planning messages in newspaper/magazines last few months, and almost three-fourths, 10,929 (74.9%) of women did not hear family planning messages on television last few months. Only, 5636 (38.6%) of women reported that they were visited a health facility in the last 12 months. Out of reproductive-age women who have visited a health facility in the last 12 months, 1935 (34.3%) had a discussion about FP with the healthcare worker and 1606 (28.5%) were counseled by healthcare workers regarding the side effects of contraceptives. Out of women counseled regarding the side effects of contraceptives, 754 (46.9%) of women were told how to deal with side effects. The survey indicated that the majority (93.8%) of women had good knowledge about any contraceptive methods (**Table 3**).

Variables	Frequency	Percent
Heard family planning on the radio last few months		
Yes	3615	24.8
No	10,978	75.2
Heard family planning on television last few months		
Yes	3664	25.1
No	10,929	74.9
Heard family planning in the newspaper/magazine last few months		
Yes	927	6.4
No	13,666	93.6
The visited health facility in the last 12 months		
Yes	5636	38.6
No	8957	61.4
Discussed FP with healthcare worker (n = 5636)		
Yes	1935	34.3
No	3701	65.7
Counseled by healthcare worker regarding the side effects (n = 5636)		
Yes	1606	28.5
No	4030	71.5
Counseled by healthcare worker how to deal with side effects		
(n = 1606)	754	46.9
Yes	852	53.1
No		
Knowledge of any contraceptives		
Good	13,686	93.8
Poor	907	6.2

Table 3.
Exposure to mass media and family planning messages among reproductive age women in Ethiopia, 2016.

4.4 Utilization of implant contraceptive methods

The magnitude of implant contraceptive methods utilization among reproductive-age women in Ethiopia was 9.4% (95% CI: 8.8, 10.0). There was a disparity of implant contraceptive utilization based on regions of Ethiopia; 212 (1.5%) reproductive age women utilized implant contraceptives from the Amhara region, and 186 (1.3%%) women utilized implants contraceptive from Addis Ababa city administration (**Figure 1**).

The overall prevalence of current contraceptive utilization among reproductive-age women in Ethiopia was 26.9%. The most preferred contraceptive method for reproductive-age women was injectable 1824 (12.5%) whereas emergency contraception 8 (0.1%)was the least preferred contraceptive method (**Figure 2**).

4.5 Factors associated with implant contraceptive utilization

In bivariate logistic regressions analysis; marital status, place of residence, educational status of women, current working status, number of living children, age at first childbirth, abortion history, fertility preference, husband desire for more children, decision making on contraceptive use, discussed FP with a healthcare worker, counseling about contraceptive side effects, knowledge on contraceptives, heard family planning message on radio, heard family planning message

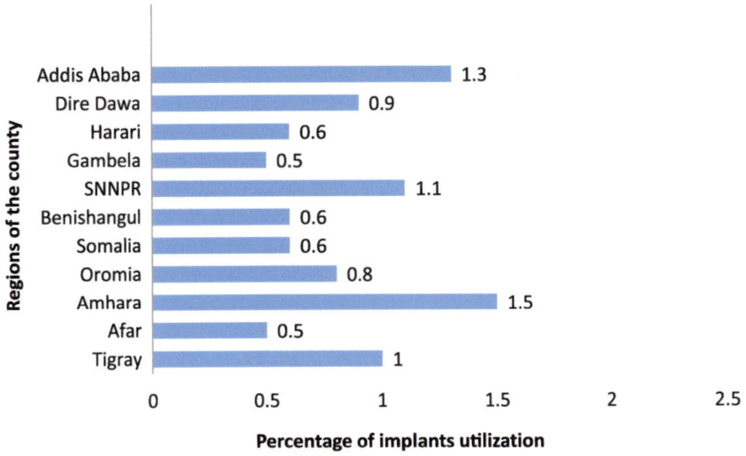

Figure 1.
Utilization of implant contraceptive methods among reproductive age women by region of Ethiopia, 2016.

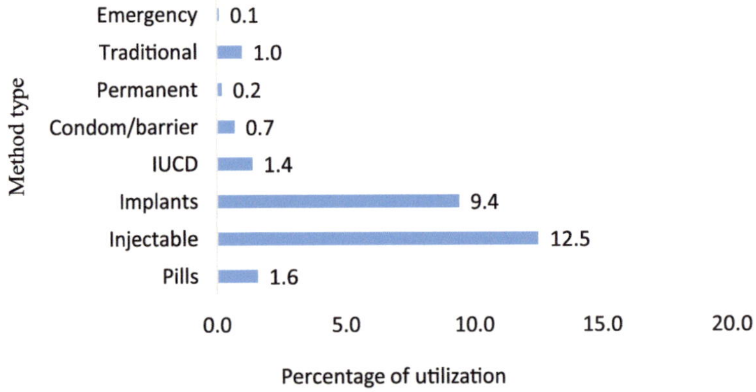

Figure 2.
Utilization of currently contraceptive methods by method type among reproductive age women in Ethiopia, 2016.

in newspaper and heard family planning message on television were identified candidate variables for multivariable logistic regression at p-value less than 0.2. Accordingly, the result of multivariate logistic regression analysis revealed that marital status, place of residence, number of living children, history of a terminated pregnancy, husband desire for more children, decision making on contraceptive use, knowledge on contraceptives, discussed FP with the healthcare worker and heard family planning message on television were significantly associated with utilization of implant contraceptives.

Married reproductive-age women were 1.94 times (AOR = 1.94, 95%CI: 1.42, 2.65) more likely to use implants as compared to those women who are never married, divorced, and widowed. Urban women were 1.66 times (AOR = 1.66, 95%CI: 1.32, 2.10) more likely to use implants as compared to their rural counterparts. Women having 1–2 living children was 39% times (AOR = 0.61, 95%CI: 0.42, 0.88) less likely to use implants as compared to women having five and more children. Likewise, women having 3–4 living children was 42% times (AOR = 0.58, 95%CI: 38, 0.90) less

Variables	Utilization of implants		COR (95% CI)	AOR (95% CI)
	Yes	No		
Marital status				
Married	1217	10,251	2.19 (1.85, 2.59)	1.94 (1.42, 2.65)*
Never married/divorced/widowed	161	2964	1	1
Residence				
Urban	456	3524	1.36 (1.21, 1.53)	1.66 (1.32, 2.10)*
Rural	922	9691	1	1
Educational status				
No formal education	826	6054	1.33 (1.07, 1.65)	0.74 (0.52, 1.06)
Primary school	311	4351	0.70 (0.55, 0.88)	0.77 (0.55, 1.07)
Secondary school	140	1825	0.75 (0.57, 0.97)	0.88 (0.61, 1.28)
College/University	101	985	1	1
Respondents' current working				
status	595	4439	1.50 (1.34, 1.68)	1.08 (0.93, 1.69)
Yes	783	8776	1	1
No				
Number of living children (parity)				
None	538	3902	1.01 (0.80, 1.27)	0.83 (0.56, 1.22)
1 to 2	573	5643	0.74 (0.59, 0.93)	0.61 (0.42, 0.88)*
3 to 4	170	2963	0.42 (0.32, 0.54)	0.58 (0.38, 0.90)*
5 and more	97	707	1	1
History of a terminated pregnancy				
Yes	151	956	1.58 (1.32, 1.89)	1.48 (1.11, 1.98)*
No	1227	12,259	1	1
Age at first childbirth				
Not had childbirth	50	268	1.40 (0.99, 1.99)	1.33 (0.79, 2.26)
Less than 18 years	693	5044	1.03 (0.85, 1.25)	1.07 (0.84, 1.64)
18–24 years	492	6827	0.54 (0.45, 0.66)	0.34 (0.24, 1.06)
25 and above years	143	1076	1	1
Fertility preference				
Wants within 2 years	297	3417	0.31 (0.27, 0.36)	0.35 (0.27, 1.46)
Wants after 2 years	273	4688	0.21 (0.18, 0.24)	0.35 (0.72, 1.12)
Wants no more children	121	2664	0.16 (0.13, 0.20)	0.75 (0.49, 1.50)
Undecided	687	2446	1	1
Does husband want to have more				
children?	986	8508	1.39 (1.23, 1.57)	0.64 (0.48, 0.84)*
Yes	392	4707	1	1
No				
Decision maker for using				
contraception	163	2084	0.17 (0.14, 0.22)	0.41 (0.59, 1.09)
Mainly respondent	742	7613	0.22 (0.19, 0.25)	0.82 (0.39, 1.16)
Mainly husband/partner	190	2889	0.15 (0.12, 0.18)	2.09 (1.27, 4.11)*
Jointly	283	629	1	1
Others				
Knowledge on contraceptives				
Good	1336	12,350	2.23 (1.63, 3.05)	9.01 (4.59, 18.90)*
Poor	42	865	1	1
Discussed FP with the healthcare				
workers	204	1731	1.01 (0.84, 1.20)	1.59 (1.22, 2.06)*
Yes	388	3313	1	1
No				

Variables	Utilization of implants		COR (95% CI)	AOR (95% CI)
	Yes	No		
Counseled by healthcare worker about side effects				
Yes	168	1438	0.99 (0.82, 1.20)	1.29 (0.98, 1.68)
No	424	3606	1	1
Heard FP's message on the radio				
Yes	255	3360	0.67 (0.58, 0.77)	0.91 (0.68, 1.20)
No	1123	9855	1	1
Heard FP's message on television				
Yes	198	3466	0.47 (0.40, 0.55)	1.60 (1.45, 2.81)*
No	1180	9749	1	1
Heard FP message in newspapers				
Yes	63	864	0.69 (0.53, 0.89)	0.92 (0.58, 1.48)
No	1315	12,351	1	1

*Statistically significant (p-value <0.05).

Table 4.
Bivariable and multivariable analysis for implant contraceptive utilization among reproductive age women in Ethiopia, 2016.

likely to use implants as compared to women with five and more children. Besides, those women who reported their husband's desire for more children were 36% times (AOR = 0.64, 95% C.I: 0.48, 0.84) less likely to use implants than those who reported that their husband would not want more children. Women who had a history of terminated pregnancy were 1.48 times (AOR = 1.48, 95% C.I: 1.11, 1.98) more likely to use implants as compared to those women who had no history of terminated pregnancy. Women who had a joint decision on contraception were having 2.09 times (AOR = 2.09, 95% C.I: 1.27, 4.11) higher odds of using implants than those who decided with the help of other persons. Women who had good knowledge of contraceptives were 9 times (AOR = 9.01, 95% C.I: 4.59, 18.90) more likely to use implants as compared with those who had poor knowledge. Women who discussed FP with healthcare workers were 1.59 times (AOR = 1.59, 95% C.I: 1.22, 2.06) more likely to use implants as compared to those women who did not discuss FP with a healthcare worker. Women who heard family planning messages on television were 1.60 times (AOR = 1.60, 95% C.I: 1.45, 2.81) more likely to use implants than those women who did not hear family planning messages on television (**Table 4**).

5. Discussion

This all-inclusive study provides vibrant evidence on the utilization of implant family planning services and associated factors among reproductive-age women in Ethiopia. Besides, the finding of this study revealed that the current utilization of implants was very low as compared to the national family planning coasted implementation targets which planned to increase contraceptive prevalence rate to 55% at the end of 2020 by increasing the share of the implant to 33% in the method mix [18]. This may imply the need to evaluate and strengthen the designed interventions like community health education and behavioral change communication (BCC) to avert attitudinal and informational barriers and misconceptions towards implants family planning methods. Moreover, the finding may also infer the poor quality of family planning counseling, especially on the prevailing myths and misconceptions of implant contraceptive methods by health care professionals. This study also indicated that the proportion of women using implant contraceptive methods was much lower than the level of use at the global level [20].

The overall prevalence of implant contraceptive utilization among reproductive-age women in Ethiopia was 9.4% (95% CI: 8.8, 10.0). The finding is almost consistent with the result of other previous studies [21–23]. However, the current prevalence is lower than the findings of other studies [24–26]. The reason for these discrepancies could be due to differences in the provision of reproductive health services, availability, and accessibility of long-acting family planning methods in safe and convenient services for all women. The variation might also be due to socio-demographic, religious belief, norm, and other cultural differences which could have a paramount effect on implant contraceptive utilization.

The current prevalence is also lower than the results of other studies done in different parts of the country [10, 27, 28]. The discrepancy might have occurred due to a difference in the study population. This study was conducted among reproductive-age women residing in both urban and rural areas, whereas those studies were conducted based on urban settings which increase the proportion of women using implant contraceptive methods.

In the current study, marital status was an independent predictor of implant contraceptive method utilization among reproductive-age women in Ethiopia. Married reproductive-age women were 1.94 times more likely to use implants contraceptives as compared to those women who are never married, divorced, and widowed. The finding is consistent with a study conducted in Nigeria [24]. This is because married reproductive age women have a higher probability of practicing regular sexual intercourse than those women who are never married, divorced, and widowed [29, 30]. Furthermore, most married reproductive age women might have the desired number of children which might have a paramount effect on implant contraceptive utilization.

The residence was also independently associated with implant contraceptive utilization. Urban women were 1.66 times more likely to use implants as compared to their rural counterparts. The finding is supported by a systematic review and meta-analysis conducted on factors associated with long-acting family planning service utilization in Ethiopia [31]. This could be because urban women are more likely to be better educated, have better access to the health care service, and better access to family planning messages through mass media than rural women which have a vital impact on implants contraceptive utilization [32]. Conversely, rural women may need more children to get help for their fieldwork which has a negative effect on their implant's contraceptive utilization [33–36]. This may imply the need to strengthen the community-based implant family planning service provision through the effort of health extension workers which could have a contribution to the increasing use of contraceptive implants by rural women.

Women having 1–2 living children were 39% times less likely to use implants as compared to women with five and more children. Likewise, women having 3–4 living children were 42% times less likely to use implants as compared to women with five and more children. The finding is supported by a systematic review and meta-analysis done in Ethiopia [31], and other previous studies [27, 37, 38]. The reason could be women with five and more children may think that the number of children that they already have could be enough for them. This may also be due to the reason that reproductive-age women having a fewer number of children may need to bear more children to attain the desired family size [39]. Additionally, women with more births would be more likely to be older and they could likely prefer a longer period of spacing pregnancies than younger women [40]. Different literature reported that utilization of modern contraceptives including implants could increase as the number of living children increases [10, 41, 42].

Furthermore, women who reported their husband's desire for more children were 36% times less likely to use implants than those who reported that their husband would not want more children. The finding is supported by a systematic review and meta-analysis done in Ethiopia [31], and other similar studies [24, 27, 37, 38]. This is attributable to gender expectations which can limit women's autonomy and the benefits that women can gain when they do a decision to contraceptive use. In most parts of the Ethiopian community, husbands' opposition could delay the decision to use contraceptives. Thus, this entails enhanced efforts in the empowerment of women as part of family planning programs [43].

Women who had a history of terminated pregnancy were 1.48 times more likely to use implants as compared to those women who had no history of terminated pregnancy. This finding is consistent with a study in Luanda, Angola, which indicated that a history of abortion was associated with implant contraceptive use [44]. The reason could be explained by those women with a history of terminated pregnancy might be had an unintended pregnancy, but they may not desire to have children currently or within a few years. Thus, to achieve their wish women may use implant contraceptives or will use long-acting methods.

Women who had a joint decision on contraception were having 2.09 times higher odds of using implants than those who decided with the help of other persons. The finding is consistent with other studies [24, 27, 37]. This indicated that the involvement of women regarding fertility and choice of contraception decision had an increased possibility of modern contraceptive use including long-term methods [45]. This strengthens evidence reported on the importance of male involvement in joint couple's decisions on family planning method choice, and contraceptive utilization [7].

Women who had good knowledge of contraceptives were nine times more likely to use implants as compared with those who had poor knowledge. The finding is supported by other studies conducted in different settings [24, 26, 27, 37]. This might be due to the fact that having a better understanding and knowledge of contraceptive methods could help women to know more about the duration of protection, advantage, safety, and side effect of each contraceptive as well as where to get the methods.

Women who discussed FP with healthcare workers were 1.59 times more likely to use implants as compared to those women who did not discuss FP with a healthcare worker. The finding is consistent with a study conducted in Nigeria [24]. This implies that counseling and informed choice are important principles in the provision of family planning services that could help women to use contraceptive methods they preferred. Furthermore, women may understand the benefit of implants over short-acting methods in its longer protection of pregnancy and convenience to use while discussing with a healthcare worker.

Women who heard family planning messages on television were 1.60 times more likely to use implants than those women who did not hear family planning messages on television. The finding is supported by a systematic review and meta-analysis done in Ethiopia [31], and other previous studies [24, 27, 37, 38]. This could be explained by the fact that women who heard family planning messages on mass media may have a better understanding and a good insight on implant contraceptives, and can compromise unreasonable misconceptions and other barriers which preclude family planning service utilization.

6. Strength and limitations of the study

The study used nationally representative data with a large sample size which better reflects the proportion of reproductive-age women using implant contraceptive method and its associated factors at the national level. The temporal relationship between implants contraceptive use and the determinant variables cannot be assured since the study used data from a single time survey, and the evidence should be utilized with caution. The analysis did not incorporate some important factors like distance to a health facility, quality of family planning services, peer-related factors that could influence reproductive-age women's implant contraceptive behavior as this is not collected in the EDHS data. Besides, the association of qualitative variables like sociocultural factors to implants contraceptive utilization was not addressed as qualitative information was not fully available in the EDHS dataset.

7. Conclusions

The study showed that the magnitude of implant contraceptive utilization among reproductive-age women in Ethiopia is very low. The finding of this study also showed that marital status, place of residence, number of living children, a history of a terminated pregnancy, husband desire for more children, decision making on contraceptive use, knowledge on contraceptives, discussed FP with the healthcare worker and heard family planning message on television were independent predictors of implants contraceptive use among reproductive-age women in Ethiopia. The finding of this study suggests any intervention strategy which is designed and being implemented to promote implants contraceptive method utilization should consider the aforementioned factors for its better success. In addition, the provision of quality counseling and information on FP, and women empowerment should be promoted so that women can freely decide on the type of contraceptive they would like to use. Moreover, emphasis should be given to rural women to implants contraceptive method use.

Acknowledgements

We thank the Demographic Health Survey Program (http://www.dhsprogram.com) for the data.

Authors' contributions

BDM wrote the proposal, analysis, report writing, and drafted the manuscript. CAW made revisions to the proposal, participated in data analysis, and drafted the manuscript. All authors reviewed, revised, and approved the manuscript for publication.

Funding

No funding has been obtained from any source to carry out this study.

Competing interests

The authors declare that they have no competing interests.

Declarations

Ethics approval and consent to participate

After developing a protocol, permission to access the 2016 EDHS data was obtained from the MEASURE DHS website at: www.dhsprogram.com by agreeing with the conditions of DHS data use stated on the DHS consent letter to the author. Ethical clearance to conduct the survey was approved by the Ethical Review Board of Ethiopia Central Statistical Agency (CSA) and the Ethiopian Health and Nutrition Research Institute (EHNRI) Review Board, the National Research Ethics Review Committee (NRERC) at the Federal Democratic Republic of Ethiopia. As indicated in the EDHS 2016 publications, written informed consent for participation was taken from study participants and written informed consent for participation was also obtained from their parent or guardian for those children (under 16 years old).

Availability of data and material

The dataset of the EDHS is not available as a public domain survey dataset but can be accessed with the request by registration on the MEASURE DHS website at: www.dhsprogram.com

Abbreviations

AOR	adjusted hazard ratio
CI	confidence interval
EDHS	Ethiopian Demographic and Health Survey
FP	Family planning
MEASURE DHS	monitoring and evaluation to assess and use results demographic and health surveys
SNNPR	Southern Nations, Nationalities, and Peoples' Region.

Author details

Birye Dessalegn Mekonnen[1*] and Chalachew Adugna Wubneh[2]

1 Department of Nursing, Teda health Science College, Gondar, Ethiopia

2 Department of Pediatric and Child Health Nursing, School of Nursing, College of Medicine and Health Science, University of Gondar, Gondar, Ethiopia

*Address all correspondence to: birye22@gmail.com

References

[1] Köngeter S, Good GL. Cultivating cultures of inclusion in social service organizations: An international collaboration. Transnational Social Review. 2017;7(3):325-330

[2] DeSA U. World Population Projected to Reach 9.7 Billion by 2050. Department of Economics and Social Affairs of United Nation; 2015

[3] EDHS E. Demographic and Health Survey 2016: Key Indicators Report. Vol. 363. The DHS Program ICF; 2016. p. 364

[4] Shah S. Determinants of human development index: A cross-country empirical analysis. International Journal of Economics and Management Studies. 2016;**3**:7

[5] Ahmed S, Li Q, Liu L, Tsui AO. Maternal deaths averted by contraceptive use: An analysis of 172 countries. The Lancet. 2012;**380**(9837):111-125

[6] Abate MG, Tareke AA. Individual and community level associates of contraceptive use in Ethiopia: A multilevel mixed effects analysis. Archives of Public Health. 2019;**77**(1):46

[7] Mustefa GTJTM, Ayalew S, Habibe S, Gudissa T. Utilization of implant contraception and factors associated among women attending family planning clinic of Ejere Health Center, Ejere Woreda, West Shewa Zone of Oromia region, 2016. Methods. 2016;**31**

[8] Kabalo MY. Utilization of reversible long acting family planning methods among married 15-49 years women in Areka town, Southern Ethiopia. International Journal of Scientific Reports. 2016;**2**(1):1-6

[9] Elias B, Hailemariam T. Implants contraceptive utilization and factors associated among married women in the reproductive age group (18-49 year) in southern Ethiopia. Journal of Women s Health Care. 2015;**4**(7):281

[10] Mohammed E, Tadese L, Agero G. Acceptance of long acting reversible contraceptive methods and associated factors among reproductive age women in Adama Town, Oromia Regional State, Ethiopia. Clinical Medicine Research. 2017;**6**(2):53

[11] Hendrixson A. Population control in the troubled present: The '120 by 20' Target and Implant Access Program. Development and Change. 2019;**50**(3):786-804

[12] Endriyas M, Eshete A, Mekonnen E, Misganaw T, Shiferaw M, Ayele S. Contraceptive utilization and associated factors among women of reproductive age group in Southern Nations Nationalities and Peoples' Region, Ethiopia: Cross-sectional survey, mixed-methods. Contraception and Reproductive Medicine. 2017;**2**(1):10

[13] Gebre-Egziabher D, Medhanyie AA, Alemayehu M, Tesfay FH. Prevalence and predictors of implanon utilization among women of reproductive age group in Tigray Region, Northern Ethiopia. Reproductive Health. 2017;**14**(1):62

[14] Ngo TD, Nuccio O, Pereira SK, Footman K, Reiss K. Evaluating a LARC expansion program in 14 sub-Saharan African countries: A service delivery model for meeting FP2020 goals. Maternal and Child Health Journal. 2017;**21**(9):1734-1743

[15] Teferra AS, Wondifraw AA. Determinants of Long Acting

Contraceptive Use among Reproductive Age Women in Ethiopia: Evidence from EDHS 2011. 2015

[16] Health FDRoEMo. Ethiopia Health Sector Transformation Plan (HSTP) 2015/16-2019/20. Ethiopia: Federal Ministry of Health Addis Ababa; 2015

[17] World Health Organization. Success Factors for Women's and Children's Health: Peru. Peru: World Health Organization; 2015

[18] Ethiopia. MoH. Costed Implementation Plan for Family Planning in Ethiopia, 2015/16-2020. 2016

[19] Meskele M, Mekonnen W. Factors affecting women's intention to use long acting and permanent contraceptive methods in Wolaita Zone, Southern Ethiopia: A cross-sectional study. BMC Women's Health. 2014;**14**(1):109

[20] United Nations. Trends in Contraceptive Use Worldwide. Obtenido de The Department of Economic and Social Affairs; 2015

[21] Aviisah PA, Dery S, Atsu BK, Yawson A, Alotaibi RM, Rezk HR, et al. Modern contraceptive use among women of reproductive age in Ghana: Analysis of the 2003-2014 Ghana Demographic and Health Surveys. BMC Women's Health. 2018;**18**(1):141

[22] Fekadu GA, Omigbodun AO, Roberts OA, Yalew AW. Factors associated with long acting and permanent contraceptive methods use in Ethiopia. Contraception and Reproductive Medicine. 2019;**4**(1):9

[23] Bikorimana E. Barriers to the use of long acting contraceptive methods among married women of reproductive age in Kicukiro District, Rwanda. International Journal of Scientific and Research Publications. 2015;**5**:513

[24] Ojo OONC, Alabi PI. Predictors of the usage of contraceptive implants among women of reproductive age in Ondo State, Southwest Nigeria. Journal of Preventive Medicine and Hygiene. 2020;**61**:E39-E47. DOI: 1015167/2421-4248/jpmh20206111367

[25] Baig D, Saleem D. Factors affecting hormonal and non-hormonal contraceptive method use in women presenting to reproductive health services-a centers of Karachi. Journal of Dental and Medical Sciences. 2012;**2**(1):8-21

[26] Anguzu R, Tweheyo R, Sekandi JN, Zalwango V, Muhumuza C, Tusiime S, et al. Knowledge and attitudes towards use of long acting reversible contraceptives among women of reproductive age in Lubaga division, Kampala district, Uganda. BMC Research Notes. 2014;**7**(1):153

[27] Bewket Zeleke L, Gella MM, Almaw Derseh H, Alemu AA, Abebe Kassahun E, Gelaw KA. Utilization of long-acting contraceptive methods and associated factors among female health care providers in East Gojjam Zone, Northwest Ethiopia, in 2018. BioMed Research International. 2019;**2019**

[28] Zenebe CB, Adefris M, Yenit MK, Gelaw YA. Factors associated with utilization of long-acting and permanent contraceptive methods among women who have decided not to have more children in Gondar city. BMC Women's Health. 2017;**17**(1):75

[29] Nyarko SH. Prevalence and correlates of contraceptive use among female adolescents in Ghana. BMC Women's Health. 2015;**15**(1):60

[30] Coll CVN, Ewerling F, Hellwig F, de Barros AJD. Contraception in adolescence: The influence of parity and marital status on contraceptive use in 73 low-and middle-income countries. Reproductive Health. 2019;**16**(1):21

[31] Dasa TT, Kassie TW, Roba AA, Wakwoya EB, Kelel HU. Factors associated with long-acting family planning service utilization in Ethiopia: A systematic review and meta-analysis. Contraception and Reproductive Medicine. 2019;**4**(1):14

[32] Kassa TB, Degu G, Birhanu Z. Assessment of modern contraceptive practice and associated factors among currently married women age 15-49 years in Farta District, South Gondar zone, North West Ethiopia Science. Journal of Public Health. 2014;**2**(6):507-512

[33] Tekelab T, Melka AS, Wirtu D. Predictors of modern contraceptive methods use among married women of reproductive age groups in Western Ethiopia: A community based cross-sectional study. BMC Women's Health. 2015;**15**(1):52

[34] Johnson OE. Determinants of modern contraceptive uptake among Nigerian women: Evidence from the national demographic and health survey. African Journal of Reproductive Health. 2017;**21**(3):89-95

[35] Adebowale AS, Gbadebo B, Afolabi FR. Wealth index, empowerment and modern contraceptive use among married women in Nigeria: Are they interrelated? Journal of Public Health. 2016;**24**(5):415-426

[36] Adebowale SA, Adedini SA, Ibisomi LD, Palamuleni ME. Differential effect of wealth quintile on modern contraceptive use and fertility: Evidence from Malawian women. BMC Women's Health. 2014;**14**(1):40

[37] Abera R, Kote M, Shegaze M, Andarge E, Hussen S. Determinants of implant utilization among married women of childbearing age in Chencha Town, Southern Ethiopia, 2017: A case-control study. BioMed Research International. 2020;**2020**

[38] Desalegn M, Belachew A, Gizaw M, Kejela G, Gudeta R. Utilization of long-acting and permanent contraceptive methods and associated factors among married women in Adama town, Central Ethiopia: Community based cross-sectional study. Contraception and Reproductive Medicine. 2019;**4**(1):22

[39] Matovu JK, Makumbi F, Wanyenze RK, Serwadda D. Determinants of fertility desire among married or cohabiting individuals in Rakai, Uganda: A cross-sectional study. Reproductive Health. 2017;**14**(1):2

[40] Anguzu R, Sempeera H, Sekandi JN. High parity predicts use of long-acting reversible contraceptives in the extended postpartum period among women in rural Uganda. Contraception and Reproductive Medicine. 2018; **3**(1):6

[41] Mohammed A, Woldeyohannes D, Feleke A, Megabiaw B. Determinants of modern contraceptive utilization among married women of reproductive age group in North Shoa Zone, Amhara Region, Ethiopia. Reproductive Health. 2014;**11**(1):13

[42] Yalew SA, Zeleke BM, Teferra AS. Demand for long acting contraceptive methods and associated factors among family planning service users, Northwest Ethiopia: A health facility based cross sectional study. BMC Research Notes. 2015;**8**(1):29

[43] Geleta D, Birhanu Z, Kaufman M, Temesgen B. Gender norms and family planning decision-making among married men and women, rural Ethiopia: A qualitative study. Science Journal of Public Health. 2015;**3**(2):242-250

[44] Morris N, Prata N. Abortion history and its association with current use of modern contraceptive methods in Luanda, Angola. Open Access Journal of Contraception. 2018;**9**:45

[45] Melka AS, Tekelab T, Wirtu D. Determinants of long acting and permanent contraceptive methods utilization among married women of reproductive age groups in western Ethiopia: A cross-sectional study. Pan African Medical Journal. 2015;**22**(1)